YOUR ARTHRITIC

CW00381608

GEORGE TARGET has b
thirty years. His many publ.
novels and non-fiction on a variety of topics, as well as
numerous articles for magazines and newspapers. He has
also appeared frequently on TV and radio. He is
married, and lives in Norfolk.

Overcoming Common Problems Series

The ABC of Eating
Coping with anorexia, bulimia and
compulsive eating
JOY MELVILLE

Acne
How it's caused and how to cure it
PAUL VAN RIEL

An A–Z of Alternative Medicine
BRENT Q. HAFEN AND KATHRYN J.
FRANDSEN

Arthritis
Is your suffering really necessary?
DR WILLIAM FOX

Birth Over Thirty
SHEILA KITZINGER

Body Language
How to read others' thoughts by their gestures
ALLAN PEASE

Calm Down
How to cope with frustration and anger
DR PAUL HAUCK

Common Childhood Illnesses
DR PATRICIA GILBERT

Coping with Depression and Elation
DR PATRICK McKEON

Curing Arthritis Cookbook
MARGARET HILLS

Curing Arthritis – The Drug-free Way
MARGARET HILLS

Depression
DR PAUL HAUCK

Divorce and Separation
ANGELA WILLANS

Enjoying Motherhood
DR BRUCE PITT

The Epilepsy Handbook
SHELAGH McGOVERN

**Everything You Need to Know about Contact
Lenses**
DR ROBERT YOUNGSON

**Everything You Need to Know about Your
Eyes**
DR ROBERT YOUNGSON

Everything You Need to Know about Shingles
DR ROBERT YOUNGSON

Family First Aid and Emergency Handbook
DR ANDREW STANWAY

Fears and Phobias
What they are and how to overcome them
DR TONY WHITEHEAD

Feverfew
A traditional herbal remedy for migraine and
arthritis
DR STEWART JOHNSON

Fight Your Phobia and Win
DAVID LEWIS

Fit Kit
DAVID LEWIS

Flying Without Fear
TESSA DUCKWORTH AND DAVID
MILLER

Goodbye Backache
DR DAVID IMRIE WITH COLLEEN
DIMSON

Guilt
Why it happens and how to overcome it
DR VERNON COLEMAN

How to Bring Up your Child Successfully
DR PAUL HAUCK

How to Control your Drinking
DRS W. MILLER AND R. MUNOZ

How to Cope with Stress
DR PETER TYRER

Overcoming Common Problems Series

How to Cope with your Nerves
DR TONY LAKE

How to Cope with Tinnitus and Hearing Loss
DR ROBERT YOUNGSON

How to Do What You Want to Do
DR PAUL HAUCK

How to Cope with your Child's Allergies
DR PAUL CARSON

How to Enjoy Your Old Age
DR B. F. SKINNER AND M. E.
VAUGHAN

How to Interview and Be Interviewed
MICHELE BROWN AND
GYLES BRANDRETH

How to Love and be Loved
DR PAUL HAUCK

How to Say No to Alcohol
KEITH McNEILL

How to Sleep Better
DR PETER TYRER

How to Stand up for Yourself
DR PAUL HAUCK

How to Start a Conversation and Make Friends
DON GABOR

How to Stop Smoking
GEORGE TARGET

How to Stop Taking Tranquillisers
DR PETER TYRER

If Your Child is Diabetic
JOANNE ELLIOTT

Jealousy
DR PAUL HAUCK

Learning to Live with Multiple Sclerosis
DR ROBERT POVEY, ROBIN DOWIE
AND GILLIAN PRETT

Living with Grief
DR TONY LAKE

Living with High Blood Pressure
DR TOM SMITH

Living Through Personal Crisis
ANN KAISER STEARNS

Loneliness
DR TONY LAKE

Making Marriage Work
DR PAUL HAUCK

Making the Most of Middle Age
DR BRICE PITT

Making the Most of Yourself
GILL COX AND SHEILA DAINOW

Making Relationships Work
CHRISTINE SANDFORD AND WYN
BEARDSLEY

Meeting People is Fun
How to overcome shyness
DR PHYLLIS SHAW

No More Headaches
LILIAN ROWEN

One Parent Families
DIANA DAVENPORT

Overcoming Tension
DR KENNETH HAMBLY

The Parkinson's Disease Handbook
DR RICHARD GODWIN-AUSTEN

Second Wife, Second Best?
Managing your marriage as a second wife
GLYNNIS WALKER

Self-Help for your Arthritis
EDNA PEMBLE

The Sex Atlas
DR ERWIN HAEBERLE

Six Weeks to a Healthy Back
ALEXANDER MELLEBY

Solving your Personal Problems
PETER HONEY

Overcoming Common Problems Series

Overcoming Common Problems

YOUR ARTHRITIC HIP
AND YOU

George Target

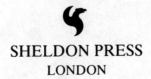

SHELDON PRESS
LONDON

First published in Great Britain in 1987 by
Sheldon Press, SPCK, Marylebone Road, London NW1 4DU

British Library Cataloguing in Publication Data

Target, G. W.
    Your arthritic hip and you.——(Overcoming
common problems)
    1. Arthritis——Psychological aspects
    2. Hip joints——Diseases——Psychological
aspects
    I. Title   II. Series
    362.1'96722   RC933

    ISBN 0–85969–518–2
    ISBN 0–85969–519–0 Pbk

Typeset by Deltatype, Ellesmere Port
Printed in Great Britain by
Richard Clay Ltd, Bungay, Suffolk

Contents

PART III *Alternative Therapies*

Introduction

During the Second World War, fighting in Italy, land of Saint Francis and spaghetti con carne, I was blasted against a stone wall by the explosion of a mortar-shell . . . and had my left hip dislocated.

It remained untreated for several uncomfortable days, until the joint was eventually snapped back into place by a friendly German medical orderly in a prisoner-of-war camp. After a slow recovery and few problems I was on the go again by the end of five or six months – with not even a scar to boast about when I got back home.

I then played football, rugby, cricket, once ran a mile in under five minutes, boxed a bit as a middleweight, collected various coloured belts at judo and karate . . . and forgot those 'battles long ago'.

Then, in my late forties, I started to get sudden twinges of pain in my left hip. Nothing much at first: the occasional spasm, increasing stiffness, a growing inability to scramble up and down the cliffs at the bottom of our garden. The twinges became jabs, and the jabs became bolts, swifter, more intense, leaving me in a sweat.

Until my wife insisted that I go to the doctor.

'Sounds like osteoarthritis,' said our local general practitioner. 'Better have it X-rayed. I'll get you an appointment.'

Those mysterious shadows confirmed the diagnosis, and he gave me the standard information: a slowly progressive disease of the joints, with breakdown of cartilage and changes in the bones, caused by wear and tear, possibly the result of injury, bad posture, or over-weight. The onset can be accelerated by occupational stresses, with coal-miners, dockers, and farm-labourers frequently its victims, and the frequency increases with age. And he gave me all manner of good advice about taking life a bit easier, not running for buses, leaving heavy lifting for other people, looking on the bright side.

'If and when it gets too bad,' he said, 'I'll put you in for the hip joint replacement operation.'

He then described this in reassuring terms, and finally made out a prescription for a hundred analgesic tablets, two to be taken every four hours as necessary.

There wasn't a lot I felt like saying.

However, on the theory that to understand what's going on is the first step to doing something useful about it, my wife and I consulted an ancient medical encyclopaedia we'd bought years ago at a jumble sale.

No known drug or injection can be relied upon as a cure, but cod-liver oil is thought by some to be capable of checking the disease if taken during its early stages. A warm, dry house, built on gravel or sand, is most desirable. Climate is of immense value, warm and sunny, but dry and bracing. It is considered that heliotherapy may have beneficial effects.

'Sun-bathing,' said my wife. 'You're good at that, so we're making a fine start.'

The waters of Bath, Buxton, Cheltenham, Harrogate or Tunbridge Wells prove helpful to some patients. For those who wish to combine a long sea voyage with a visit to a Spa where adequate treatment may be obtained, nothing could be better than a spell at the wonderful hot baths at Rotorua in New Zealand . . .

'That's for me,' I said. 'A warm, dry, desirable residence on gravel or sand at Rotorua.'

'Always merry and bright,' said my wife. 'We can't lose!'

But that battered old book was a beginning, and we subsequently wandered far and wide (and often got lost) in the medical undergrowth of established facts and contradictory opinions, venerable ideas and original theories, drugs and diets and treatments and dubious therapies. However, I emerged with considerable information about how to live with an arthritic hip – and now have one new metal-and-plastic hip joint.

So if you've had any of those first nasty twinges, then perhaps I may be able to help you.

I've been cared for by doctors, nurses, surgeons, physiotherapists, and several other sorts of therapist. And I have listened to them, learned, and sometimes even argued.

I have assumed that anything helpful anybody can tell us about how to ease the pain of an arthritic hip, and even cure it, ought to be shared among sufferers. So I have accepted advice and information from both orthodox and alternative sources: standard textbooks, medical publications, popular paperbacks, health magazines, newspaper articles, and folk wisdom.

Here, then, is a collection of ideas I've found helpful, and if this book adds anything useful to the stock of common knowledge I'll be delighted. But please remember that it's not about arthritis in general, merely about osteoarthritis: in particular about osteoarthritis of the hip-joint, how to live with it, the various treatments, and possible cures. And it most certainly isn't a substitute for the advice and care of your doctor, more a helpful supplement . . . because the more you know, the better you'll be. And sooner.

PART I

Living With Your Arthritic Hip

1

A Burning Pain in Your
Hip Joint

What is arthritis?

The first indisputable fact I discovered was simple.

As with most such medical terms, the word 'arthritis' doesn't mean any more than its literal translation from Greek into English.

'Doctor,' you say, 'I have a burning pain in my hip-joint.'

There follows the taking of your symptoms and medical history, an examination, perhaps some tests, even an X-ray . . .

'Yes,' says your doctor, eventually, 'I'm afraid you've got osteoarthritis.'

Which only means in Greek exactly what you said in English: *osteon,* a bone, plus *arthron,* a joint, plus *itis,* an inflammation or inflammatory disease . . . with 'inflammation' deriving from the Latin *flamma,* a flame.

All your doctor is really saying is that you've got a burning pain in your hip-joint.

To know the truth in plain English takes the mystery out of your condition, which I believe is reassuring — because fear of the unknown is the enemy of healing. So, wherever possible, I intend to use everyday words rather than the pedantically correct medical terms.

The second indisputable fact is that there is no single disease called arthritis, but a collection of various distinguishable conditions — well over a hundred.

Few of these are supposed to be curable by orthodox medicine, though it's always possible to relieve the symptoms, minimize the discomfort, and reduce the damage and disablement. In the case of an arthritic hip-joint you can prevent further deterioration. There's no need to become even a partial cripple.

Hope is important: give it up, and you might as well give up altogether. Where there's life, even in the worst case, there's the promise that you'll soon be walking normally again.

What causes the disease?

Another fact is that there's no generally accepted single cause, but almost as many theories as there are medical schools.

According to some it's merely a condition of age: the longer you live the more likely you are to suffer from it.

All creatures with bones experience degenerative changes in them if they survive long enough, and almost every human feels the effects of these changes by the age of fifty or sixty. You slow down, and can't run for the bus or climb the stairs.

True, many people are old and out of their depth in a mortgage at thirty, and a few stay young and healthy until the day they die. But otherwise it's the classic paradox: medical science preserves us from diseases which used to kill us in youth, and we now live into middle-age to become victims of diseases which they can't yet prevent or cure: we are protected against pneumonia, meningitis, or typhoid . . . only to die from cancer or cardiac arrest.

Or to develop arthritis.

A combination of factors?

Some believe it to be caused by a combination of factors: an inherited predisposition, or perhaps a genetic weakness, which is then activated by an infection, or a self-indulgent lifestyle, bad or inadequate diet, unhealthy environment, chronic fatigue, stress, emotional tension, even spiritual distress.

And, of course, an accident may chip or crack the surface of a joint, or a fracture may alter the alignment of its bones with each other, and this damage may precipitate deterioration.

A hip, I discovered, is more likely to develop osteoarthritis if it has been dislocated — particularly if it was damaged when being set or returned to its socket. Which was the partial explanation of my own case.

Years of being over-weight may also be one of the possible causes, or slack posture, hard manual labour, or excessive preoccupation with strenuous sports such as football, gymnastics, or long-distance running, even standing for hours as an assistant in a shop . . . any prolonged muscular strain. And remember that most mothers work physically harder than most men: cooking, cleaning, shopping, looking after children.

8

How you live, then, the demands you lay on yourself and others, your expectations and ambitions and unfulfilled desires, what you eat and how you work. All of these factors can either provoke your arthritis or worsen it.

However, on the same basis of understanding, if you change your lifestyle for the better, modify your demands, acquire different expectations, reconsider the true value of your ambitions, do something creative about your desires, eat and drink more sensibly, work at a human rhythm, march to another drum . . . you can make peace with yourself, and live without arthritis.

An excess of acids?

Again, according to some, osteoarthritis is caused by an excess of specific acids in the body. If we maintain a balanced diet, and thus neutralize these acids as we absorb them from our food, there's little problem — except that a lot of the food we are sold these days lacks natural balance, isn't fully nourishing, and so we are undernourished in the midst of apparent plenty. After years of such inadequate eating our body carries too much toxic acid, which is circulated by the blood, distributed in the muscles, and deposited as small gritty crystals on the bones and between the joints. And these crystals cause wear to the working surfaces, swelling, and consequent pain.

Gout is the best-known type of arthritis admitted by nearly every researcher to be caused in this way, the excess being that of uric acid — usually believed to be brought about by too much rich food and strong red wine. Food may not be the only factor involved, as various metabolic and hormone disorders have also been detected, along with inherited abnormalities — and even drugs taken for other conditions may often trigger the agony.

Types of joint

Two main types of joint are liable to arthritis.

Some are extremely flexible, with a wide range of complicated movements: shoulders, wrists, fingers, and feet. And some have to carry the weight of your body, and so must be load-bearing and stable, as well as being capable of simpler movements: hips, knees, and ankles.

We shall concentrate on the hip-joint.

The hip-joint

The hip is an ingenious ball-and-socket joint, with a ball on top of the femur (thigh bone) held in a deep socket at the side of the pelvis.

Femur is Latin for thigh, and *pelvis* is Latin for basin, and the whole arrangement of bone can be seen as a basin-like structure in which the lower intestines are held.

Both the surface of the ball at the top of the thigh-bone and the interior surface of the socket are covered with a thin layer of *cartilage,* which is a tough gristle, white and smooth — the word 'cartilage' is derived from the Latin for gristle. And the whole joint is sheathed in a strong elastic membrane, the *capsule* — from the Latin for a 'little case' — which in turn is lined with a thinner membrane, the *synovium,* which gets its name from the fact that it produces *synovia,* a term invented by Paracelsus, a sixteenth-century Swiss occultist and physician to describe what he though was a fluid which nourished several parts of the body. It is now used by doctors solely to name the fluid of the joints.

The capsule helps to hold everything together, and is filled with synovial fluid, which resembles the white of a raw egg, and is the lubricant that ensures the smooth sliding of the ball in its socket. At the ends of the various surrounding muscles are the tendons which attach them to the bones, and there's also a system of small blood vessels which bring nourishment to the whole structure.

When healthy these bones and muscles move easily, and the cartilage works as a shock-absorber, with the lubricating fluid keeping everything working with the minimum of friction. It's a strong joint, surrounded by the powerful muscles of the thigh and buttocks, so any defect soon becomes important. Yet, for all its strength, the working surfaces are strangely vulnerable to arthritis. And, because the sheath and linings are rich in nerve-endings, when these become inflamed the joint is not only difficult to move but also desperately painful.

However, please remember that your body is a self-supporting system: when a part is infected or injured it works to resist the infection or repair the damage.

Your hip-joint is no exception.

Arthritis in the joint

What, then, happens when the joint is affected by arthritis?

To be pedantic, the word 'arthritis' should only refer to inflamed joints, and these inflammatory conditions ought to be distinguished from conditions of ordinary wear-and-tear. It is incorrect to call wear-and-tear of the bones by the word for a burning pain in the joints, osteoarthritis — though, obviously, the two conditions often exist together. The proper medical term is *osteoarthrosis*— with *osis* being the Greek for condition or state: the word then meaning a condition of the joint, especially if diseased.

But I'll use the more familiar term.

There are two main types of these inflammatory diseases which can affect your hip: *rheumatoid arthritis,* a condition of the muscles, and *osteoarthritis,* a condition of the joints.

The word 'rheumatoid' derives from the Greek *rheum,* to flow. In the late Middle Ages this was used to describe any excessive watery discharge from the eyes or nose.

To have rheumatism, then, or to be rheumatic, originally meant to be subject to such an abnormal flow, or 'defluxion of rheum'. The concept behind this was the ancient notion that our health depends upon four bodily fluids or 'fluxes' known as the 'four humours' — phlegm, blood, choler, and black bile. If one of these gets out of correct balance, or 'fluxes' more copiously than the others, then you are 'out of humour,' ill at ease, ill, or dis-eased.

Since the Middle Ages the word 'rheumatism' has come to mean a disease of the muscles, usually having an effect on the joints surrounding them, characterized chiefly by more or less severe pain — 'rheumatoid' thus means having the characteristics of rheumatism.

Rheumatoid arthritis

In rheumatoid arthritis there is inflammation of the muscles, the pain of which causes restriction or alteration of movements to avoid or ease the discomfort. The joint is thus subjected to positions and stresses it was never intended to withstand, the cartilage starts to wear away at these new points of pressure, and eventually cracks or disintegrates. With the already painful muscles pulled slightly out of position, the tendons loosen, and the whole joint slackens. Movement is then even more impaired, and the process of deterioration seems to feed upon itself, with the pain getting worse and worse.

Osteoarthritis

In osteoarthritis, probably one of the severest and most disabling forms of arthritis, there isn't much inflammation of the muscles to start with, but small cracks appear in the cartilage, which get deeper, and it simply crumbles and wears away under the pressure of the body's weight. An X-ray examination will reveal some loss of cartilage at the point of maximum stress, between the upper surface of the ball on top of the thigh-bone and the inside surface of the socket in the pelvis. So, whatever the cause, it's obviously a degenerative disease.

It usually affects the larger weight-bearing joints, and is a wear-and-tear condition which develops in joints subject to heavy strain or injury. Sometimes only one joint (such as the hip) is affected, and pain is confined to that area. The bones roughen, and the synovial membrane creases into thick folds. Fibrous tissues and new bone form around the weight-bearing surfaces of the joint, and, gradually, movement becomes limited to avoid pain. This leads to further disuse and the wasting of the muscles, and this in turn increases the stress on the joint. If the condition progresses, the joint surfaces grate on each other and become so worn that they often fuse, and bony *ankylosis* occurs — the Greek for a condition of stiffness.

To sum up: not all, but most arthritic hips are probably cases of wear-and-tear as you get older, with the cartilage covering the facing surfaces of the joint gradually crumbling away, or the degeneration is brought about by other factors. There is considerable friction, grating, soreness, and inflammation. Not surprisingly, the result is increasing pain and worsening stiffness.

2

Signs to Look For

The condition can be controlled, eased, the process of deterioration reversed — the disease even cured.

If left untreated the condition will obviously get worse, and the damage done to your hip and your life may well harden beyond all possible treatment or repair. But if you start doing something positive and practical as soon as you notice any of the signs and symptoms, then you've got nearly everything going for you. And the sooner you begin to take notice of your body, and what it's trying to tell you, the better it will be.

All of us have occasional twinges of pain in the joints, and it's easy enough to imagine that a slight ache is the first symptom of some fearful disease.

Remember the narrator of *Three Men in a Boat* who 'idly turned the leaves' of a medical textbook in the British Museum, 'glanced' at a list of 'premonitory symptoms', and discovered that the only disease he *hadn't* got was housemaid's knee?

His cure was beefsteak and beer every six hours, one ten-mile walk every morning, bed at eleven sharp every night, and the advice 'not to stuff up his head with things you don't understand'.

So, yes, be interested in your body, take care of the works, listen for the music of your feelings, learn your true needs and natural rhythms — but don't ever be dominated by mere flesh and bone. Life is more than keeping a finger on your own pulse at all hours of the day and night, and there are many more useful activities than collecting bottles for your medicine cupboard.

Balance is the secret of more than arthritis.

Warning symptoms

As a rough and ready guide, twinges that don't last long are probably only twinges — but if you get even a few hours of pain in your hip, any swelling, and certainly any stiffness, it's better to see your doctor.

The onset is usually gradual, and you'll probably experience a dull ache more than a sharp pain, which will persist and begin to drag and get you down, feel worse after exercise, and much better after a rest.

Sometimes your *sciatic* nerve may be affected — a Greek word which means 'pertaining to the hips.' It's the largest nerve in your body, extending from the lower part of your spine, through your buttocks, and down your thighs into your legs. If it's compressed or becomes inflamed you'll have shooting pains and numbness in your hip and along the shin of your affected leg.

There are several signs to watch for:

- Increasing difficulties with your hip, obvious pain and any stiffness of movement, limitation or distortion of its rotation.
- Flexion, or your ability to bend, may remain comparatively good for some time, but the awkward posture which ensues is generally shown by an increased lumbar lordosis and tilting of the pelvis. 'Lordosis' is the Greek for a forward curvature of the spine, usually in the lower back.
- A spasm of intense pain when you try to move your whole leg a little further in any direction than you can normally bear.
- Atrophy of the thigh muscles is common — *atrophy* is the Greek for wasting — so your leg may seem to be losing its old strength, even getting visibly thinner, and you may have cramps in your calf, or start ricking your ankle.
- Feeling more tired than you used to, if you're losing weight without dieting, or simply don't feel like eating.
- Feeling you're strangely depressed, or rather more emotional, shorter-tempered — even 'out of humour'.
- Sometimes you'll be free from pain, and start to wonder whether or not you're making too much fuss about nothing, but other times you'll feel as if you're on the rack.

These symptoms may disappear for a week, or months, even years perhaps, and then return: sometimes they may disappear permanently.

But why take chances?

Go to see your Doctor

It's obviously best if you take notice of the first symptoms early, and start some form of treatment before the disease gets beyond simple remedy. Prompt diagnosis will reduce the chance of future pain and possible disability, yet may sufferers tend to belittle their symptoms, and postpone going to their doctor for months, even years . . . by which time the damage has been done.

So if you believe that you have any of these early signs, then please go to your doctor at once. If you're mistaken, nothing has been lost except a little of your time — but if you're right, then you've made a good start.

When we reach the age at which we're likely to develop these symptoms of osteoarthritis, most of us are concerned about our health. Having to go to the doctor at all is probably a bit worrying, and when we're worried we tend to get anxious, possibly a touch forgetful.

It's a good idea, then, to note down a brief description of what you've felt about the behaviour of your hip, no matter how trivial the details. What might seem unimportant to you may make a lot of difference to the correctness of the diagnosis and the helpfulness of the treatment. Moreover, it will save your doctor's time.

For example, tell the doctor about any close relatives with similar problems, and be ready to answer questions about your previous illness or injuries, your work, the sports you play, and the tablets or medicines (if any) that you are already taking. There's probably a full record on the files, but there's also nothing like your own words for the casual remark which might reveal a significant clue to the condition of your hip.

Listen carefully to everything you doctor tells you: all the details about the drugs being prescribed, how many tablets to take at a time, and when . . . all the advice about ways and means of relieving the pain and making your life easier. And make notes, don't trust your memory. Your doctor won't mind in the least, and will probably regard you as a model patient. And a good relationship can do nothing but improve your chances.

Treatment
Unfortunately orthodox prognosis does not hold out much

radiant hope — *prognosis* is the Greek for a prediction or forecast of the course and termination of the disease. Osteo-arthritis is a degenerative condition, and, therefore, any treatment given is unlikely to produce a cure. All that can reasonably be expected is some remission of symptoms. Though there is a glimmer of light. Bearing this strict limitation in mind, treatment is surprisingly successful.

Standard treatment is directed to the relief of pain and the accompanying disability, and generally consists largely of physiotherapy, the prescription of analgesic drugs (*analgesic* is the Greek for 'rendering insensible to pain') and, in advanced cases, surgery is recommended to replace the damaged joint with an artificial one.

So it's essential that your doctor has an informed interest in arthritis, knows about recent advances in research and some of the latest treatments, or is at least willing to refer you to a specialist.

Above all, your doctor must be sympathetic. If you're merely told that you're getting on in years and can expect the occasional twinge, then change your doctor. As a private patient this is your paying privilege, and even on the National Health Service you are entitled to make such a change. In either case the doctor may not like it — but it's *your* arthritis. For unless you and your doctor respect each other, *you'll* be the one to suffer the needless pain. You must be regarded as a whole person, not just as a patient suffering from a disease.

Yes, there has to be the best possible clinical treatment for the pain and stiffness of your hip joint — but there must also be full consideration of your anxieties and fears, because few factors are more important than the maintenance of psychological balance under the stresses imposed by arthritis.

3

Breaking the Circle
of Depression

Successful treatment largely depends on your own attitude, because negative emotions such as hopelessness and anxiety can be as destructive as the disease.

Arthritis only affects your bones, but despair can corrode your whole being. So you must be positive, take a creative part in the process of healing, do everything you can to bring about an improvement in your condition, encourage your responses to the treatment, admit your fears, cherish your hopes, and talk freely to your doctor and friends — but most of all to your family: wife or husband or lover. And don't forget that children are members of the family: people need love, and loving them is good for you.

No drug is so potent as love, no therapy can work on your body without involving your emotions, your intelligence, and your spirit. Summon up these, and you'll increase your own capacity for self-healing.

Depression and Anxiety

Depression is most excellent fuel for the inflammation of arthritis. So dampen down your depression, and starve the inflammation of unnecessary fuel. Break the circle . . . it hardly matters where.

If the sun is shining, your pain seems less, and the absence of pain enables you to enjoy the sunshine. So you either start with the day being lovely because you haven't got any pain, which will help to keep the pain under control, or you start with the absence of pain, and this will help you to enjoy the day even more — which will also keep the pain under control.

To be happy is to be on the way to healing, and to be active is to work against stiffening.

But, with all that said, it's still worrying to know that you've got an arthritic hip.

How much worse will you get? Are you heading for a wheelchair? Will your job be kept open for you if you have to take time off. How long is it going to last? What is it going to do to your marriage? Suppose you have to be admitted into hospital for the hip joint replacement operation? What's the success rate? How will you manage afterwards? Where will the money come from? What about the mortgage?

These natural anxieties seem part of the disease, with the condition of your hip causing the anxieties, and the anxieties making the condition that much worse.

But once this is understood you can break that circle, your anxieties are easier to control than your arthritis. True, it's just not possible to stay cheerful all the time. You simply wouldn't be human if you didn't lose your heart every so often. But if you let it all get you down too far, too often, you'll stay down. Slump in a chair feeling miserable for too long, and you'll stiffen into the final immobility — not merely of limbs, but of despair.

Accept the fact that you've got an arthritic hip, that it's now as much a part of you as your healthy one. But also accept the fact that you can *choose* to have them both healthy instead of both diseased.

Choose health, decide that you're going to do everything you can to live more fully, even learn from the most painful lessons — and you've started your own cure.

Dealing with your depression

The best way to reduce anxiety and relieve depression is to talk about it all with somebody you trust: doctor, family, friends, neighbours — or even a stranger. You'll find most people willing to listen, if only you give them a chance to tell you about *their* troubles — and troubles shared are troubles eased.

Sympathy and understanding are healing qualities, and you will help your own healing by understanding the needs of others, and being sympathetic towards them.

Whatever you do, don't suffer in silence. For silent suffering can curdle the milk of human kindness. Yes, you must have courage . . . but a stiff upper lip prevents you smiling, and a smile will help to dissolve more than the problem of your own stiffness:

18

'A merry heart maketh a cheerful countenance, and doeth good like a medicine: but by sorrow of the heart the spirit is broken and a broken spirit drieth the bones.'

And it's your bones with which we're concerned, especially when the lubricating fluid doesn't work, and your hip joint dries out.

If you start feeling sorry for yourself, you'll end by having even more to be sorry about: self-pity will destroy you quicker than arthritis.

A psychosomatic disease?

It's perhaps too much to claim that arthritis may be a psycho-somatic disease. *Psychosomatic* is a compound of two Greek words, *psyche,* the soul, and *soma,* the body: meaning that a trouble in your soul can cause a disease in your body. But it's undoubtedly true that it often starts after a time of both emotional and physical stress: a death in the family, a divorce, an accident, shock, the loss of your job, an apparently unrelated illness, or there may be resentment, repressed anger or hostility, personality clashes or conflicts.

These psychological factors do not necessarily cause the disease, but they often precede it, and certainly tend to make it worse.

In other words, your deteriorating hip-joint may not have just happened to you for no good reason, but is possibly the result of prolonged stress which has so exhausted your body's reserves that its normal functions are impaired.

It may be hard to admit to yourself that you aren't happy, that perhaps there's something wrong with your marriage, or that you're seething with unacknowledged anger or frustrated desires. Or perhaps you feel that your ambitions are never likely to be realized, that you're being defeated by life, losing touch with your dreams, or perhaps you feel a sense of guilt or shame or inadequacy, despise yourself for what you are.

All of these feelings can lead to stress.

Not that all stress is bad for you: it can often be exhilarating. The tension you feel before the big occasion actually helps you to perform better. And when you cease to be excited you cease to feel at all.

But being stuck in a traffic-jam with a train or plane to catch can cause a tension we should all do without . . . and prolonged tension of any sort is better avoided.

Try relaxing

Test yourself: the next time you're feeling angry or frustrated or under stress, notice how tightly you're clenching your fists or hunching your shoulders, perhaps even tensing your whole body. And watch out for restless movements, fidgets, finger tapping.

All of these are obvious signs of inner tensions. Try to relax your body: unclench your fingers, lower your shoulders, release the tight muscles of your chest and abdomen, fold your hands loosely in your lap, smile. The smile will spread inwards: you'll feel the gentleness welling up. A few quiet breaths, and you'll be at peace with yourself and your world . . . breathing is the simplest balm for stress.

Try it: if you do find yourself under a strain, then stop whatever you're doing, take a deep deep breath, hold it for as long as it's comfortable — don't attempt to beat your own record, you're not swimming under water . . . then breathe out slowly. Lower your shoulders, let yourself go limp, stay loose. Breathe in again, deeply, . . . then breathe out, making sure that you're still loose, and relaxed.

And then start your life again, more slowly, breathing easily.

Try auto-suggestion

Don't neglect the apparent simplicity of auto-suggestion.

Dragging yourself around muttering that you're feeling terrible can't possibly do you any good, while to tell yourself that you're feeling better can't possibly do you any harm.

The classic formula is to repeat this well-known sentence every morning before getting out of bed and every night before dropping off to sleep: 'Each day, and in every way, I am getting better and better.'   It may be simplistic, but does everything have to be complicated?

Improving your environment

It's a good idea to give some attention to where and how you live. Just as you know how good you feel when you're clean and rested, so a clean and restful room will help you feel equally good. It's refreshing to change your shirt or your dress, or alter the style of your hair: so why not refresh yourself by giving your room a change round?

It's not necessary to fit an expensive wall-to-wall carpet, nor put up new wallpaper — though either would work all manner of psychological wonders, but try another way of arranging the furniture, or have a bowl of roses or sea-shells, or paint the door spring green or autumnal orange . . . or you could make or buy a few bright covers for the old cushions, or even new curtains if you can afford them.

What about two or three cheerful posters? or the photograph of a person or place you love? the reproduction of a serene landscape by Constable? a vision of Venice by Turner?

Try shaded lamps: find a balance between light by which you can read, and a warm glow. Or what about a dimmer-switch so that you can adjust the brightness to suit your mood?

Try indoor plants, all those beautiful colours and shapes — not only a pleasure to look at, but interesting to grow.

Try little bowls of herbs or flower-petals. Yes, it's all a question of taste, but let it be your own taste rather than the passive acceptance of what's already there.

Loving yourself

Give you own life the same respect and consideration that you give to others. Yes, 'love your neighbour as yourself', but you have to love yourself to start with. How can you reach out to others if you aren't standing firmly on your own psychological legs?

So be aware of your own deeper feelings and needs when you begin to crumble around the edges under pressure, especially when you'd prefer to be on your own. Sometimes you'll enjoy other people's company — but why not enjoy your own occasionally? Yes, there are times for parties and fun and games and loud music . . . but there are also times for solitary walks and thoughts 'too deep for tears'.

It's not always possible to be the happiest of good companions if you're in pain, so why not be sensible and excuse yourself?

'Sorry, but my hip is hurting rather badly.'

No, you're not playing for sympathy, but you will get it.

4

Living with Pain

The function of pain

Pain is a necessary signal from our body that all is not well, so to suppress it may not always be good for us — because unless we receive the warning we may never know that anything is going wrong until it is too late.

If your hip is painful, and you ignore it, grit your teeth and push yourself to the limit, you'll only generate further pain, and almost certainly damage your joint even more.

The 'threshold' of pain, the moment when it becomes too much to bear without some sort of grimace or other reaction, varies widely from person to person. Some people cry, some merely shrug, one person may hardly notice an injection, another may faint. Religious and political martyrs have been tortured to death . . . and their smiles have mocked their torturers.

Your body has got the capacity to experience pain, and yet not to give in to it, not let it dominate your life. We can in fact learn to use our mind to modify the effects of even the severest pain, though sometimes the circumstances have to be a bit larger than ordinary life.

A boxer, charged with adrenaline, can fight on with a broken nose or fractured knuckles, taking punches which would flatten you or me. Long-distance runners break through what they call the 'pain-barrier' to finish the last lap in a glorious burst of speed. A soldier with a dislocated hip can still manage to dive for the nearest cover.

When you have to, you can — somehow.

Don't be ashamed of pain

The extent to which you feel pain, how far you allow it to interfere with your life, depends as much upon you as it does upon the actual severity: what sort of a person you are, what inner resources you've got, your circumstances, even how you're feeling at the time.

But you are the only judge of your own pain. So please don't ever be ashamed to admit that your hip is hurting, because you're not morally responsible for your body's unique threshold or ability to resist. Besides, it's merely a less than human tradition of our society that we're 'supposed' to bear pain without protest.

Never ignore what your body is telling you.

'The great object of life,' wrote Byron, who lived to the full despite the pain and deformity of a club-foot, 'is to feel that we exist, even though in pain.'

How *do* you live with the pain and awkwardness of an arthritic hip-joint?

Drug treatments

Well, there's not much virtue in scourges and hair-shirts, and little need to endure pain for the mere sake of doing so.

If you need drugs, take them. But be guided by the doctor you trust, take the smallest amount possible, and remember that most drugs have side-effects, so be careful.

Also remember that drugs are usually prescribed to lessen the effects of your *symptoms*: they do not necessarily cure what is a chronic degenerative disease.

Causes matter as much as symptoms.

There are hundreds of thousands of people suffering from one or more of the various types of arthritis, dozens of drugs are currently being prescribed for their treatment, and most patients are persuaded that they need to go on taking them for months and years.

That means the drug companies make vast profits, and so have a vested interest in the pushing of their products. Various drugs have therefore been pushed with what some doctors have called 'unjustified enthusiasm'.

A recent example is Opren. When it was first promoted it was described by its makers as a 'major breakthrough' in the treatment of arthritis, with only 'mild and transient side-effects' . . . but soon there were reports that in fact it had 'potentially dangerous' effects, and that some patients had actually died after taking it. Eventually, after a lot of pressure, it was withdrawn.

So do please be careful: whatever the drug, there are usually side-effects. Some are minor and temporary, but some can be damaging and permanent.

Never disregard the possibility of adverse reactions to any drugs you may be prescribed — why take chances with your own health?

If you experience any sort of unexpected effects, such as a headache, or dizziness, or a sore throat, indigestion, nausea or vomiting, a rash, or a fever – *anything at all* — then tell your doctor at once. The dosage can be reduced or another drug prescribed.

And be scrupulously careful about the drugs: never more than the dose, never more often than stated. If you're to take the tablets *after* meals then don't take them *between* meals: it may not sound a vital distinction, but it could make all the difference as to whether or not you suffer intestinal bleeding.

Types of drugs

For a fuller and much better qualified discussion of possible drugs please consult your doctor, but, briefly, there are three main categories used in the treatment of arthritis.

- Analgesic (Greek for rendering insensible to pain.)
- Drugs which reduce the inflammation and swelling.
- And those which act to alter the process of the disease rather than merely ease the effects of its symptoms.

Analgesics

Analgesic drugs control, or at least relieve, the pain.

Some powerful yet highly dangerous analgesics, such as morphine, can ease it almost completely — but these are addictive, with terrible long-term results. So less harmful drugs have been developed: non-addictive, fast-acting, and with fewer side-effects.

Among the first of these was *aspirin*, and it's still the most commonly prescribed. It suppresses pain, and usually reduces inflammation — but in high doses causes loss of appetite,

24

digestive troubles, ulcerative colitis, stomach and intestinal bleeding, nausea, vomiting, ringing in the ears, and mild deafness. You also need to take it every few hours, so it can be expensive, and it's mostly prescribed in tablet form.

With so many side-effects to aspirin, many other pain-killers were developed — including *paracetamol*, which is increasingly prescribed. But *never* take more than the recommended dose, as it can cause anaemia (blood deficiency), cyanosis (blueness of your lips and skin), and damage to your liver and kidneys.

Because of the almost inevitable irritation caused to the lining of the stomach by most of the stronger drugs in this category, such as *phenylbutazone*, *indomethacin*, and *naproxen*, these are often prescribed as suppositories. These are small soap-like pills which you insert into your rectum or vagina, where they are absorbed by your body without having to pass through your stomach or intestines.

Incidentally, it's best to avoid those handy aerosol cans of pain-relieving spray as used on footballers to deaden the effects of a kick. True, you don't feel the pain in your hip for quite a long time afterwards but don't be deluded into thinking that your arthritis is going away. The mere absence of pain, however welcome, doesn't necessarily mean that all's well.

Recent research has also indicated that many analgesics used to control arthritic pain and inflammation may, in fact, hasten the process causing the symptoms.

Professor Dennis Lowther, of Monash University, Melbourne, using an electron microscope, has discovered that cartilage is a 'network of protein fibres impregnated with a molecular gel', or jelly. This jelly is the lubricant, 'normally renewed every eight days or so'. But 'certain antiarthritic drugs' actually 'decrease the manufacture of replacement gel', thus 'increasing the friction' between the surfaces of the joint.

Your doctor will know the details, or can find them in the medical literature, and the information may influence any decision about your future treatment.

Drugs to reduce inflammation and swelling

There are many drugs to reduce the inflammation and swelling, and they are used more in the treatment of rheumatoid arthritis than for an arthritic hip joint.

25

The most famous (or notorious) of these are the *steroids*, which, when first marketed, were promoted as 'miracle' drugs. They are extremely efficient, but, precisely because they are so powerful, they can also cause indigestion, gastritis, blood pressure, skin eruptions, bruising and swelling of the face and body, excessive hair-growth, and even mental disturbance. There's also evidence that they can affect the mineral content of bone — hardly a recommendation for the treatment of a crumbling joint. For these and other reasons they are now prescribed with extreme caution, usually in much smaller doses — with consequent reduction in the unpleasant side-effects.

They are often injected directly into the affected joint, which means that they start working immediately where they're most needed — again with a consequent reduction in the side-effects. The area will be cleaned with an antiseptic, you'll be given a local anaesthetic, and your doctor or a specialist will inject a solution of the drug. Distinct improvement will probably follow three or four days later and may last four or five months, with further injections as necessary.

Drugs which alter the disease process

Finally, there are drugs which alter the process of the disease. Again, these are used more in the treatment of rheumatoid arthritis. They are extremely powerful, and have many serious side-effects: interference with the production of blood-cells, the working of the kidneys, muscle weakness and fatigue, skin rashes, and diarrhoea. They are usually a last-ditch resort, when everything else has failed to control the pain and stiffness, when there's progressive disability and damage to the joint.

Gold salts and *penicillamine* are the most commonly prescribed, gold salts by injection, and penicillamine by mouth. Nobody is quite sure how they work, but they do seem to arrest the progression of the disease in some people. It may take two or three months for the effects to be noticed, during which time you'll need to have regular blood and urine tests.

Take sensible precautions

Whatever drugs you are prescribed, do please take them exactly as directed. Don't ever take any non-prescribed medicine at the same time without telling your doctor — you may be mixing a dangerous cocktail.

And remember that most drugs don't mix well with alcohol, so don't wash down your tablets with anything stronger than water, milk, or light lagers.

Some drugs are used merely for the suppression of pain and the relief of stiffness, so if the pain has gone, and you're no longer stiff, *then stop taking them* — but first ask your doctor to make quite sure.

It's also worth making sure that you aren't being used as a guinea-pig without your permission. Many doctors participate in clinical trials of new drugs sponsored by drug companies, and are paid to report on their effectiveness. However, if you are being used to test a new drug, your doctor has a clear moral responsibility to explain this to you, and you have the right to refuse.

Other forms of treatment

But your doctor is more than a mobile prescription-pad, and there are all manner of other ways to control pain and treat disease than tablets.

For example, if you're constipated, more fibre in your diet, a few potatoes baked in their jackets, or replacing steam-cooked white bread by home-made wholemeal, will be much better for you than any laxative.

So, likewise, a little thought will often prevent the pain before it starts.

Vary your activities as much as possible during the day, don't spend too long doing any one thing, mix movement with frequent short rests. Find the balance between proper rest and necessary exercise: if you don't rest you'll put too much of a strain on your hip, but if you rest too much you'll stiffen and suffer pain.

So avoid standing or walking for more than 20 minutes without having a short rest — five minutes will be enough. Take the weight off your legs by sitting or even lying down.

Avoid stretching too far, don't go in for much bending from the hips, and climb or descend stairs as though you've got all day.

No need to crawl around feeling sorry for yourself — merely observe care and caution. Plan your life so that you have to bend less: keep your socks and underwear in top drawers, use a long-handled broom instead of a brush and dust-pan, and perhaps move your bed to a room downstairs.

Even the way you stand or walk or sit may have an effect: sensible shoes, a good posture (erect without being stiff), a comfortable chair, could all make the difference between pain and pleasure.

If you're sitting in your favourite chair, and start getting twinges, then move to another chair for a little while. Give your leg a change of position, and yourself another point of view.

To sit for hours watching television is to ask for trouble. Quite apart from the programmes, which may tend to create frustrations and induce stress, to be still for so long will make for stiffness. Get up out of your chair every twenty or thirty minutes, stretch your legs, walk about a bit. If possible, get somebody to massage your hips and legs at the end of the viewing session — a pleasure in itself, as well as a relief.

However, with such a persistent discomfort as arthritis, the amount of pain is no real guide as to what to do about it: again, it's really up to you, but all you've got to do is think about something else entirely.

Fill your mind with other thoughts than your hip grating away in there: beauty, happiness, pleasure, new ways of enjoying life, day-dreams, memories . . . even what to expect for tea.

One of my greatest pleasures is swimming naked in the sea, and I would imagine the beach, the sand and pebbles underfoot, the sun and the sky and the high clouds and the gulls wheeling inland, the air cool to my flesh, the waves rolling up the shore to meet me, the exhilarating shock of the water . . .

Discover your own healing day-dreams, live to the full, in your mind, in your body, in your own feelings and emotions, and there'll be less room for pain.

Mind over matter

But suppose, for whatever reasons, that none of this works.

Then study your pain, feel it, give yourself up to the whole experience, understand what's happening.

It will almost certainly ebb and flow, become more intense, and then ease . . . return . . . ease . . .

Once it seems to have reached its miserable worst, you then start thinking the tide back: it can't last for ever at that intensity, so help it recede by observing the process.

Then ask yourself why your hip is playing up just now. What have you been doing? Sitting or standing too long? Have you twisted round too suddenly? Tried to lift some heavy box or bag? Is your bed too hard or too soft? Are you cold, tense, or irritable?

Whatever the cause, do something practical about it.

Locate the pain, precisely. Visualise the exact place — and here a little knowledge of the look and shape and position and movements of the hip joint would be useful. Any textbook of anatomy has pictures, or perhaps your doctor could show you an articulated skeleton. If you see the ball and socket, the cartilage, the surfaces, the muscles and tendons, you can imagine it all moving . . . smoothly.

Put your finger on the site of the pain. How extensive is it? Where does is spread? Could you say how big it seems to be? What shape is it?

What colour would you call it? Some pains are sharp acid-green, some are bright throbbing red, some are sullen brown, bruised purple, or dreary grey, or burning orange.

What is the pain trying to tell you? That it's now getting very serious? or is just a reminder that it's still there?

Decide its intensity on a scale of ten: two, and hardly worth bothering about? Five, and getting to be a nuisance? Seven, and rising towards being unbearable.

You'll find that visualizing it in this way will lessen its effects, and may even ease them altogether for a time. Because in thinking about it so carefully you're actually thinking about what it *is*, rather than what it's doing to you.

In fact, some people use the process of visualization as a means of self-healing: they see the joint slowly restoring itself a little every day, moving more and more freely, the pain receding further and further.

Another way of using your imagination to cope with pain is to visualize your body as a castle which is being attacked by an enemy: the outer walls are breached, the troops are clambering in, but your own defenders are rushing to the place, trying to throw them back — and the fighting is the pain. When the enemy has been defeated, the fighting will stop — and so will the pain. Then you can start to rebuild your walls.

This is a vivid way of describing what's going on in your body: infection is being fought by your various natural defence systems, and to visualize them at work is to encourage the process of defence and recovery.

Don't forget the simple hot and cold compress: neither can cure arthritis, but they can certainly relieve the pain.

Soak a clean towel in cold water, squeeze it dry, and apply it to your hip until it feels numb. Then do the same with a towel soaked in hot, not boiling, water. And having somebody do it for you will be an added pleasure.

To sum up: in general, please remember that fear of pain will probably bring it on and worrying only make it worse. So don't give fear a chance: fill your hours with love and beauty and joy, give yourself to others, look at flowers and trees and landscapes and sunsets, listen to the birds and music and the laughter of children. Live each day as though it's the first day in the rest of your life, and your arthritic hip will soon be yesterday's bad news.

5

Dieting Can Help Your Hip

Some doctors still maintain that what you eat doesn't make a great deal of difference to arthritis, but even they will readily admit that to be over-weight with an arthritic hip is a serious disadvantage. Why carry about more weight on your suffering joint than you need? Every extra pound makes your day more difficult.

Try an experiment: weigh out a stone of potatoes in a sack on the bathroom-scales, and lug them up and down the stairs a few times, or ask the butcher to let you see a fourteen-pound lump of yellow fat. Either should convince you.

Arthritis is a wearing disease, and the tension of even minimal pain can leave you tired — so you must eat a well-balanced diet, with enough vitamins and essential minerals. Most doctors would allow that the inevitable ageing process, in which our bones get thinner and more brittle, can be alleviated by eating adequate proteins, and making sure that we get enough calcium.

But if you're over-weight your hip joint is under a strain it could do without. So to lose that weight sensibly, and keep it off, will make a great difference to your chances of recovery.

Losing weight

There are two main ways to lose weight: increase the physical work and amount of exercise you do without eating any more food, or eat less.

But for your body to use food faster than you're eating you'd have to be a coalminer, a ballet-dancer, or an athlete — all somewhat difficult with an arthritic hip.

This leaves eating less: reducing your intake of food to below the present wants of your body — to what it needs rather than what you fancy. You will thus oblige your body to use your stored fat — and you'll lose weight. It's important, though, to lose it *gradually* . If you reduce your intake too dramatically your body will start to 'eat' tissue. Gradual loss doesn't play havoc with your

31

metabolism. As Geoffrey Cannon says: 'dieting can *make* you fat.'

The only problem is to change your habits.

It's a bit like trying to stop smoking: lots of smokers manage it again and again, The difficulty is *staying* stopped.

Changing your eating habits

Most of us probably eat for quite the wrong reasons: we eat food that merely looks and tastes good because it's been chemically coloured and flavoured, or food that's been extensively advertised. We eat at fixed times whether we're hungry or not, or we eat because other people are eating, or because we want comfort or reassurance. We may have put on weight because of the enforced idleness of having an arthritic hip, or we might be bored and be eating too many snacks for the sake of something to do . . . and so on: food as a substitute for happiness.

The strategy, then, is to eat what you need, not what other people expect you to eat. Change your habits, and only eat what is good for you, when you need to, and in smaller amounts.

You'll have to be firm with yourself and everybody else within yards of the kitchen.

'Don't you like my cooking any more?' may demand an outraged mother or wife. 'You used to devour my chocolate cream-cake!'

However, there are a few simple tactics you can try.

- Only eat when you are hungry. To eat for any other reason than hunger is self-indulgence, or compensation for the lack of some other satisfaction. You're trying to do something about your painful arthritic hip, remember? Stop using food as a crutch.
- When you do feel hungry, drink a cup of weak tea or black coffee, or have a bowl of thin soup — even a glass of water. This will make you feel full without filling your stomach with too many calories.
- Or eat a little treat about thirty minutes before your main meal: an apple or orange to take the edge off your appetite.
- Insist on smaller portions than usual, and eat small meals regularly rather than big meals every now and again.

32

- Eat raw salads, firm fruits, and nuts — all of which need a lot of chewing. They're not only good for you, they'll slow you down — perhaps even make you tired of eating.
- Concentrate on what you're eating, taste what you put into your mouth. Chew every mouthful before swallowing, savour the flavours and textures. Don't drink much until you've finished the meal, or you'll dilute your gastric juices and not get the most from the food.
- Don't eat if you're upset or angry, as that will invite the pain of indigestion to join the pain of your hip.
- And don't try to read at the same time as you eat, and give yourself a rest from radio and television. Make the meal a happy social occasion, talk about your day and your doings. All this will help to take your mind off your hip, as well as ease the weight from it.

But please remember that you're changing the habits of a lifetime, so don't expect an immediate miracle.

6

Exercise Can Help Your Hip

Any acute arthritic hip joint must be rested from time to time, especially when it's too painful for you to do much else — but as soon as the pain lessens you must then resume gentle exercises to keep as mobile as possible. This means putting your hip through the full range of its movements several times a day — every hour or so if you can. Joints that are rarely moved through their full range usually stiffen, and are likely to be painful.

All the simpler forms of exercise, then, are even more vital to the arthritic than they are to most people.

Get out into the fresh air and free sunshine, walk on grass rather than on hard pavements or roads, move your muscles, breathe in deeply, enjoy your body. Don't overdo it, don't strain or force yourself, merely keep as active as you can. And don't walk too far away from home — remember that you'll have to walk back.

Get to know when your hip needs exercise, and when it needs rest. Too much of either can cause pain — so it's a matter of judgement and moderation. Whatever you do, don't strain or stretch too far, don't grit your teeth to finish at no matter what cost: there's no gold medal to be won. However, an ache is not yet pain, so don't stop too soon. Listen to your body: it will tell you when to stop.

In general, try to keep yourself supple — which is as much an attitude of mind as a condition of your body.

- Avoid sudden or awkward movements.
- Don't stand for too long in one position, but keep moving, no matter how slightly.
- Don't bend to pick up anything from the floor, but kneel on one knee to keep your spine upright.
- Never let anybody do for you what you can do for yourself, except, perhaps, as an occasional gesture of love and concern — as, for example, when your beloved bathes and pampers you with warm towels. It may take more time to struggle on with your socks and shoes, but it will help you not to become psychologically dependent on others.

If you enjoy gardening, there's every reason why you should continue. In moderation this is healthy exercise. Watch the old hands, who work steadily, little and often rather than in one mad rush. Use long-handled tools, don't crouch over the weeds, but kneel on a soft pad or kneeler-stool with grips for getting up and down — and always keep your back straight. Don't try to shove loaded wheel-barrows, and leave heavy weights for others.

The fresh air will do you good, the sun is a blessing, contact with the earth and the seasons will be a balm to your soul, and the growth of living things will remind you of the healing process you are encouraging.

In fact, any hobby, whether it involves movement or not, will be more than merely creative: carpentry, book-binding, dress-making, drawing and painting, clay-modelling, weaving — all will keep you active, interested in life, too fulfilled to feel miserable.

But, as with gardening, don't strain to do too much all at once.

Standing, walking, sitting

Few movements could be more simple than standing, and yet many of us tend to get it wrong.

It's been said that 'you don't stoop because you're old — you're old because you stoop.' Look at the stoopers around you who are old before their time. If we start the wrong way we are likely to go on being wrong. Simply maintain an upright posture, preserve your muscular strength, and thus keep your bones free from unnecessary stress.

When you stand, keep straight without strain. Hold your head high, reach up as though it's a balloon floating on your neck. Keep your abdomen in, but not tensed, no slouching on one hip, but balanced to distribute your weight. Every so often take a slow series of deep breaths, as many as you like, because one of the reasons you need a good posture is to enable you to breathe properly with fully opened lungs. But even when standing you are not a statue, not static, so don't remain rigid.

When you walk, keep erect without strutting, swing your arms loosely, feel free . . . and don't stride out. This is a human animal walking, not a storm-trooper route-marching into battle. Take your time, there's no hurry. Enjoy your movements.

When you sit, don't slouch into the chair, but keep your head up, shoulders straight, abdomen in, your feet flat on the floor. Choose an ordinary chair with a hard seat and an upright back, rather than a lounge recliner — which may feel more comfortable at first, but often turns into a padded rack.

Incidentally, twenty minutes in an old-fashioned wooden rocking chair will nearly always ease an aching hip or lower back, and it's a soothing activity whether you're aching or not. But make sure that the regular creaking and rocking doesn't irritate other people.

Deep breathing

The simplest of all exercises is probably the best: controlled deep-breathing several times a day — preferably in the fresh air, or at least an open window. Few of us actually take more than shallow breaths, consequently our lungs are under- used, and we become sluggish.

Stand naturally, your arms loosely by your side, take a deep breath, fill your lungs to capacity . . . then breathe out as much as you can.

Never hold the breath, but draw it in and ease it out in a continuous flow, neither stopping when your lungs are full nor empty. And breathe in through your nose rather than your mouth.

Take ten of these breaths — feel them doing you good — they will help you to feel more calm and less prone to anger, easier with yourself and the world.

Hip exercises

All of these exercises will loosen the joint, but they'll also improve and correct your posture, increase the flow of blood, strengthen your heart and lungs, and stimulate the contractions of your muscles and thus help to eliminate toxins and waste. So they'll be good for you in general.

It's important to maintain the rotation of your hip joint,

otherwise it may seize up. If your hip is already stiff, at first these movements will be restricted, but regular exercises will gradually ease the joint and loosen the muscles, your mobility will increase, and there'll be less pain.

The way you exercise is equally important: the good quality matters more than the mere quantity.

Do them every morning and evening — best of all when you are warm and relaxed from a bath or shower. Wear loose and comfortable clothes, as few as possible — none at all if you enjoy nakedness.

Try to extend the range of the movements a little more every day — but go gently, or you may do more harm than good. The test is this: if your hip-joint aches for a few minutes after you've finished, then that's about right, but if it aches for ten minutes or longer, then you've been overdoing it.

Repeat each movement a few times to start with, say three or four, increasing the repetitions day by day to about twenty.

The purpose of the exercises is to put your hip joint through its own natural movements, slowly, deliberately, with perseverance and pleasure.

But if ever you feel even the least bit dizzy, stop at once, and tell your doctor before you start them again. In fact, if you have any doubts at all about whether or not you are fit enough for even these undemanding exercises, please consult your doctor before you start them.

Now for the exercises.

- Stand behind a firm chair, hold the back as a support, and carefully swing your affected leg sideways as far as it will go without hurting too much to bear. Keep your other leg straight, and your body upright, or you'll get little benefit: don't let your body lean away from your affected leg, because then your good hip is doing all the moving — which is easier, yes, but a waste of time and effort.
- Stand by the side of the chair, hold the back as a support, and swing your affected leg backwards and forwards, keeping your body upright to avoid bending in the wrong place. This free movement without weight will help your walking.

For the next exercises you'll need to lie on your back, on the floor rather than a soft bed. A folded blanket will make it more comfortable, but you really do need the firm support rather than a yielding mattress.

- First, merely lie there for a few minutes, as relaxed and as slack as possible, Feel the floor beneath you, allow the weight of your body to be supported, to sink into itself, to become weightless and floating. Be still, and enjoy the stillness.
- Stretch and straighten your legs, curl your toes tightly, uncurl them, and then relax. Repeat, and relax.
- Stretch and straighten your legs, rotate your feet to the left, then to the right, and relax. Repeat and relax.
- Bend your left knee up towards your chest as far as you can, using both hands to give a gently sustained pull. Hold for a few seconds, and feel the muscles working and easing. Then slowly stretch your leg out straight again, and relax. Do the same with your right leg, and relax. Repeat and relax.
- Lift your left leg, keeping your knee straight and your thigh braced. You don't have to get it very high at first, just enough to clear the floor. Hold while you count to ten . . . lower slowly, and relax. Do the same with your right leg, and relax. Repeat and relax.
- Keep your heels together, and bend both knees up towards your chest as far as you can without using your hands to pull . . . and then part your knees outwards as far as they'll go. Count to ten, close your knees, and then slowly stretch your legs out straight again, and relax. Repeat and relax.
- Lift your left leg, keeping your knee straight and your thigh braced, and move it slowly to the side as far as it will go. Count to ten, move the leg to the centre, lower it, and relax. Do the same with your right leg, and relax. Repeat and relax.
- Now lift both legs, knees straight and thighs braced, and part them to the sides as far as they'll go. Count to ten, bring them together again, lower, and relax. Repeat and relax.
- Lie on your left side, and lift your right leg as far as it will go, keeping it straight. Count to ten, lower, and relax. Repeat and relax. Then turn over, do the same with your left leg.
- And, finally, turn over onto your back again, and relax in the same way as you began, feeling the support and the stillness, and enjoying your body.

These lying-down exercises can be done in the bath, which will be of great additional benefit because the warm water will give you that little extra 'lift' and enable you to relax even more.

If you can get to a warm pool occasionally this will be even better for you, because almost any exercise in water will soothe stiff muscles and help damaged joints to work more easily. Merely stand with the water up to your neck, and gradually flex yourself all over . . . or float on your back . . . or swim with a gentle but wide breaststroke, opening and kicking your legs, making them work. In fact, swimming will work small wonders on your hip, as all of its movements will be supported by the water and yet you'll be free and easy, able to enjoy yourself.

More specialized exercises

The advice of a physiotherapist is essential for any more specialized exercises than those of this simple programme. Your stiff hip involves many different muscles, so detailed knowledge of their inter-relationships and a study of your own individual needs will obviously be required for a comprehensive series of exercises intended as part of your treatment by a doctor.

Physiotherapy can't cure your arthritis, nor have much effect on the actual bones of your hip — but it most certainly improves the power and tone of your muscles. So it's well worth attending sessions if you can.

Under supervision you'll exercise in all sorts of ways: using weights and benches and bars, slings suspended from the ceiling, frames and chairs and stands. At first sight the place may resemble a torture-chamber — but please don't be put off. Those people in white coats will soon make you welcome, and you'll be feeling benefits before you know it.

Apart from the exercises there are many other pleasures: the gentle stimulation of wasted nerves and muscles by means of soft electrical pads, the application of relaxing heat by hot towels and infrared lamps, careful manipulation and massage of your hip and leg, and various forms of water therapy.

From personal experience I can say that, quite apart from the healing good they do, all these therapies can be intensely enjoyable.

Infrared lamps

You don't need to attend sessions to enjoy the warmth and comfort of a 250 watt infrared reflector heat-lamp in your own home. They're reasonably cheap, and are ideal for relieving the area immediately around your hip.

The maker's instructions will be in the box: but, briefly, you take off enough clothes to clear the site, lie comfortably on a bed, and arrange the lamp to glow two or three feet from your skin. Then give yourself up to the comfort and pleasure. But don't use it for longer than 15 minutes at most, or you might burn.

As you get better at your exercises, and perhaps become less self-conscious about your body, you may care to go in for slow, free, and unstructured dancing, preferably in the open air, best under the sun, wearing as little loose clothing as possible . . . naked if you prefer.

Go for self-expression, allow your bones to speak to you, your flesh to sing.

Perhaps your arthritis may have been caused by the denial of your body, perhaps you've been too rigid for too long . . . perhaps you haven't listened to the whispers of what it's been trying to tell you, and are now being shouted at.

But what possible harm can a little happy dancing do to any body?

7

How to Relax

Stress as a factor

There's little doubt that prolonged stress can worsen the pain of
your hip so it seems sensible to do all you can to ease your
tensions. Even in trying to avoid pain you tense your muscles,
and this can put the joint under the very pressures that cause the
pain. So it's important to relax, to have times when you loosen
your muscles and rest your mind.

Some stress is obviously inevitable: we live in the twentieth
century. But peace and quiet are still to be had once you learn
how to achieve them. You can't do much about the lunacy of the
contemporary world: but you can create a cell of sanity and
gentleness within it. Even the ordinary pressures of life, with
buses to catch and work to do, can affect your hip in several ways,
and rushing all over the place certainly won't do it much good —
quite apart from the undoubted link between tension and
arthritis.

Learning to relax

Try to rest each morning and afternoon, not for hours or you'll
get too stiff for your own good — but, say, for twenty minutes.

Give yourself this time in a warm and quiet room where you
won't be disturbed. By day close the curtains, by night turn out
all but one shaded glow of a lamp. Take off your shoes, undo a
few buttons. Settle in a deep comfortable chair, or, better still, lie
on your bed.

Then tighten all the muscles in your body. Feel the tension,
know what it's like, want to get rid of it.

Let you toes and feet go limp, allow your calves and thighs to
slacken, breathe slowly and easily, sink into the chair or the
mattress . . . now your fingers, hands, arms, shoulders . . .
experience the slackening, the loosening, first the chest, then the
abdomen.

Be patient and gentle with yourself, listen to the noises of life outside your head, the clock ticking, distant traffic.

Feel your head settling into the pillow.

Calming your mind

The calming of your mind is more difficult than the simple relaxing of your body, but worth the necessary patience.

Your body will happily respond to happy thoughts, your muscles will relax as your mind relaxes . . . and the negative of pain can be cancelled by the power of positive thinking. But it's a two-way feedback process. Because the mind will also respond happily to a happy body, your thoughts will move more slowly as your muscles loosen into rest.

Go with the flow . . . 'Ride the horse the way it's going.'

Stay with your body a while . . . but slowly change your dreams, organize your fantasies, choose your own inner delights. Start with the memory of some recent happiness: a day in the country, that holiday on the coast, an act of love and laughter. See yourself in beautiful places, feel the warmth of the sun, the coolness of the breeze, hear the many voices of the sea, smell the perfume of flowers or food cooking, float in clear green water, watch the fish sliding by like illuminated jewels.

Fill your mind with images of happy pleasure, indulge your most secret desires, coax your ideal self out from the shadows.

Once persuade your mind, and your body will respond as though the landscape of your imagination is real. You can be on holiday for as long as you like every day with your hip gradually improving.

Now come back slowly, open your eyes, look around at the room, listen to the clock, the distant traffic . . . experience your body again, move your muscles . . . think about getting up.

You'll certainly feel more relaxed and serene afterwards, and, as you get better at it, you'll be able to unwind with less conscious effort.

And, eventually, you'll be able to enter the peaceful landscape of your mind whenever you need: on the bus, in the train, waiting at the wrong end of a queue, any time, any place.

Living in the real world

Another way, completely different, to slide out from the trap of worry and compulsive thinking is to look around you at what is there: see the real world, listen to its sounds, touch it, smell it, taste what you're eating and drinking, experience everything, feel the truth of your emotions.

Move your focus from inside your head to your body, from your thoughts to your experiences. Leave your private world, and consciously join the real one. Live in the present. The past is the past, the future is yet to come . . . *this* minute is all you've really got for sure. Time is too short for wasting.

Start to express your feelings directly and with deliberate self-awareness. Don't unload them on others, but don't cripple yourself by repressing them. When you experience a feeling, express it: laugh, cry, be tender, be angry.

You don't have to go off on an ego-trip, or hurt people. Merely express your truth with gentle love. Don't blame others for what you are, but accept full responsibility for yourself. Give yourself your own permissions. Refuse to live on a licence granted by other people's opinions.

Try anger

Many doctors and therapists agree that to drag unresolved anger around with you is to be damaged by it. Arthritis is only one of the many diseases known to be affected by such psychological stresses.

So learn to discharge your anger, don't let it go sour inside you. Release the pressure before the damage is done.

But don't necessarily vent it there and then, and not always on the immediate cause. It could be more damaging than it's worth to blast your beloved, your child, your friend, or your employer, so get away to where you won't be disturbed, some place where you can make a noise . . . and let go.

Feel your anger, throw a tantrum, punch a pillow, swear if it does you any good, enter into your emotions, use your strength . . . and in a little while it will all start to feel easier, even silly or embarrassing.

If making a noise will disturb or worry other people, try

strangling a towel, silently: roll it into a rope, and twist and twist, gritting your teeth, giving it all you've got. Then release your verbal aggression by biting it hard.

Take as much time as you need to empty yourself of the anger. You'll know when to stop. Then feel it draining away, and you'll be easier — probably a bit embarrassed.

A few deep breaths, and you're back with life again.

Now, calmly, examine the causes of your anger. What was it really all about? How much of it was your fault? How were you threatened by what was said or done? Do you actually feel unloved or unwanted by the person you were angry with?

You'll probably come to see that anger is hardly ever worth what it does to you. So don't allow anybody to have that sort of power over you.

Remember that *people* don't make you angry — you give *yourself* permission to become angry. But also remember that to release positive emotions is as therapeutic as the repression of negative emotions is damaging.

So express pleasure, smile when you're happy, tell your beloved of your love, say the words, hold and cherish for all the world to see, embrace the experience.

Bodily awareness

Be aware of your body. It has a wisdom of its own. Be tender and sensitive to it. Don't wait for pain or pleasure to remind you that you've got a body. Live in the present, enjoy everything you do, use all your senses.

Massage

Massage has been called 'passive exercise', and few exercises or treatments can relieve the pain of an arthritic hip with more benefit and pleasure. It will tone your muscles, stimulate your digestion, strengthen your heart — and lead to a feeling of relaxation and peace.

'The secret,' says Sharon Kretzmer, 'is that it is so simple to do. Everybody already knows how to do it. There is nothing to learn. All we have to do is arrive at the state where we know and trust the wisdom in our hands and simply let them guide us. We step into the river and float, and the name of the river is love.'

So anybody ought to be able to give a simple massage for pleasure. You merely stroke and rub the person all over gently, using warmed perfumed oil to make it easier, doing whatever comes naturally . . . kneading, loosening, easing, flexing, rolling, shaking, even slapping. You pay special attention to the affected part, and to the face, the hands, the feet . . . treating the whole person with love and care.

Wait a couple of hours after a meal, and make it an act of celebration. Do it in a warm room where you won't be disturbed, have a little quiet music, take off your clothes, and lie on a bed or a divan, or even on the floor with a folded blanket beneath you, and give yourself up to the lavishing care of your partner. Accept the pleasure, feel what's happening, experience your body. Make sure that you aren't lying in a draught, and that the movements aren't sudden or tense.

There are all manner of linaments and embrocations on the market, almost any one of which will ease pain. Choosing is probably a matter of memory, and the evocative smell has no doubt got a lot to do with it. Wintergreen or almond oil are as good as most, and certainly cheaper than many brand-name products. You can also make your own. Add a few drops of any aromatic essence you fancy, say lavender or your own favourite perfume, to any light vegetable oil or body lotion. And remember to use it warm.

The linaments and embrocations work by causing mild inflammation of the skin, which slightly increases the surface circulation of the blood. But be careful, because some of the more old-fashioned varieties can be virulent on tender skin. Test before you start, and avoid using any of them on or near the genitals.

Apart from the reassurance of a massage by a loving partner, a qualified practitioner will be able to do so much more for you, using all manner of strokes and pressures, creating deep friction around your joints and along your spine, easing tension in your back and neck and shoulders, and perhaps even correcting the faulty posture which might be causing some of your problems.

So 'step into the river and float . . .'

Baths containing Epsom salts

There are few more relaxing therapies for stress, few better remedies for pain, than a bath containing Epsom salts before bed.

Have the water as hot as you can bear it — though *not* if you've got high blood pressure or a weak heart. Add a pound of Epsom salts, but no soap or bath-cubes. Keep the hot tap trickling to maintain the temperature. Get used to it first, then move your hip-joint gently, bending your knee, and rotating your leg. Give yourself 15 or 20 minutes, then dry yourself thoroughly, and get straight into a warm bed. Don't hang about or expose yourself to cold. Keeping warm is important. You'll sweat, but this is good. The idea is to eliminate acid or toxic wastes through your pores, so wear thick pyjamas to absorb the sweat.

In the morning have a shower or a sponge-down to wash away these wastes, and you'll be surprised how refreshed you feel.

Start with two baths a week, and make it more often as you begin to enjoy the benefits. You can vary the treatment by using sea-salt instead of Epsom salts, or mixing them half-and-half. And if you want an exhilarating experience, try adding a teaspoon of ordinary powdered ginger — but then be careful to keep the water out of your eyes and ears.

John Rowland, a consultant herbalist who for many years has run a successful clinic specializing in arthritis, recommends that a massage of the whole spine and the affected hip with oil is of great therapeutic value after such a bath. He specifies Rowlo Oil, a heady blend of ten aromatics, including juniper, clove, almond, and wintergreen, which can be bought from any good health shop or herbalist. But do keep warm, and get into bed as soon as possible.

8

The Importance of Sleep

The natural process of birth and death goes on for life. Our body is wearing out and renewing itself all the time. By day we are using our resources faster than we can restore them, and by night in sleep we recharge ourselves ready for the morning. So it's essential that we sleep well: not necessarily for any fixed number of hours, but that we get *enough* sleep of a satisfying and refreshing quality.

However with an arthritic hip you are less likely to sleep well or soundly. Almost any worry will keep you awake, and you now have the niggling thought of perhaps being eventually crippled laid like a dragging weight on top of the actual pain. If you lie too still, you'll suffer stiffness, and if you keep shifting around to avoid the pain, you'll *never* get to sleep.

Even tossing in bed worrying about not sleeping will merely cause you to sleep more fitfully. So what's to be done?

Sleeping pills — if you must

The easiest and least useful way out is to ask your doctor to prescribe some sleeping tablets.

By all means take the prescribed sedatives if you really and truly can't manage without them — but try to avoid these chemical aids to sleep: they're habit-forming, and lead to physical and psychological dependence. Accept them as a *short-term* remedy in an emergency, but understand that they're like a bandage on a broken leg: better than nothing, but not a proper treatment of the underlying condition.

Natural sleep is harder to achieve, but worth every thought and effort.

Natural aids to sleep

With sleeplessness, as with so many of our troubles, change for the better rarely comes by a dramatic breakthrough, but usually by a series of new understandings and small steps.

Broad advice is easy: 'Buy a water-bed' or 'learn how to control your mind' — but there's no simple trick.

Quietness, warmth and the satisfaction of basic human needs are obviously much more likely to make for sleep than noise, cold, and frustration.

Getting the bed right

On the assumption that your hip is stiff enough to make bending painful or difficult, you can make getting in and out of bed a lot easier by raising it on four bricks or sturdy wooden blocks — though be sure that they're standing steady. You don't want to be wobbling off at half-past two in the morning!

The mattress must be soft and giving enough for comfort, but firm enough to support your weight without sagging. Few pains are worse than an arthritic hip combined with an aching back.

A double bed with another person might be too much for both of you, because what might be snug for your partner may well be a wicked rack for your hip, and your sleepless tossing won't exactly make for the other's sweet dreams. So try two single beds side by side. If you can afford it, there are even separate single mattresses with different degrees of firmness that can be zipped together on a double bed. Either way you'll still be in loving contact — which is vitally important for both of you, because the warmth of love is the greatest healer. Yet neither of you will disturb the other's most precious sleep.

Useful guidelines

- The easiest way of being ready for sleep at night is to get up earlier in the morning.
- Another way is to be physically tired — which is where your regular exercise will be more useful — and a short walk in the open air just before going to bed will be a clincher.
- Learn how to unwind at the end of the day. Some people read an undemanding book, some listen to music, or even watch television — though if violence bothers you it's sensible not to watch most late-night programmes. And for the same reasons it's best to steer clear of too much excitement, too many arguments, chess problems, crosswords, or any strenuous mind-stretching — because the more active your brain, the harder it will be to get to sleep.

- A warm bath is a natural prelude.
- To go to bed at a regular time every night is better than at different times, so establish a pattern. Live by your own inner sense of timing, and you'll be in harmony with your own rhythms.
- Even if you smoke, try not to go to bed on a cigarette, because nicotine stimulates the nervous system and raises the blood pressure, neither of which will soothe you to sleep.
- Alcohol will undoubtedly knock you out as quickly as most sleeping tablets if you drink enough, but it has disadvantages of its own: you'll have a disturbed sleep, which will leave you tired, probably with a hangover, with no appetite for breakfast.
- It's not a good idea to go to bed hungry, but a heavy meal doesn't necessarily mean a heavy sleep, and hard-to-digest snacks of pork-pie and pickles are usually followed by rather hectic dreams. So stick to cereal and milk if you feel empty. And a warm milky beverage can induce restful sleep.

Extra comfort

- Be warm in bed: the Spartan life has its virtues, but freedom from pain isn't one of them. So don't despise bed-socks, hot-water bottles still have their uses, and an electric-blanket is the easiest way to snuggled warmth.
  However, do be careful not to slip into sleep with a hot water bottle against your flesh, because you risk being burned. Wrap it well in a towel or slide it out of the bed when you're comfortable.
- And if you wear night-clothes, warm them first.
- The gently monotonous sounds of the distant sea will encourage sleep. We can't all move house to the nearest coast, but, if you have a tape-recorder, you could record your own sound effects. Or listen to some of the tapes on the market: all manner of natural sounds and music are available, some specifically intended to ease you into sleep.

Positioning yourself for sleep

You can't sleep if your body is still tight with the tensions of the day, so being in the most comfortable position for both rest and sleep is important.

Lie straight to start with, flat on your back, with a soft pillow or no pillow at all. Keep your knees and hips straight, arms and hands by your sides. Be stretched, but not tense. Have the bed-clothes loose rather than tucked-in neatly — a continental quilt is ideal.

You can get temporary relief from the pain in your hip by putting a cushion or another pillow under your knees — but don't do it for long or too often as you may find your hip setting into the position and hard to move. And don't ever go to sleep like that, because the pain of movement in the morning won't be worth the earlier comfort.

If you prefer to sleep on your side, make sure that your pillow is bunched under your head so that your neck is as straight as it would be when you're standing.

Move your affected leg from time to time to keep it flexible, gently, as far as it will go without discomfort. And don't worry about going to sleep in any one position: you'll move naturally during the night.

Love as sleep therapy

What better prelude could there be to a deep and restful sleep than making love? Even with an arthritic hip, there's no reason at all why you shouldn't continue to enjoy a richly satisfying sexual life.

All you have to do is to go on talking with your partner, telling, listening, communicating. Given love and happy willingness to experiment, all manner of positions and variations are delight-fully possible. Any illustrated sex manual will provide lots of exciting ideas.

It is absolutely essential that you should both do everything you can to keep up the joys of life and love together. Arthritis can have a depressing effect on even the happiest marriage, because once you allow pain and inconvenience to slow you down you're in danger of stopping completely. And if full intercourse is occasionally impossible because of some temporary spasm of immobility, loving consideration will find all sorts of gentle ways to soothe and relieve sexual tensions.

Go on accepting each other, understanding — please go on *communicating*. Love is much more than the expression of physical sexuality, though any act of affection is to be welcomed. But respect and consideration for the other person as a human-being are just as essential. Arthritis is literally a wearing-out disease, but, with two people working at it, you can both find ways and means of laughing and loving.

What's one arthritic hip between two lovers?

Think positively

However, no matter what else you do to charm sleep, calm your mind as you close your eyes. Don't merely try to stop the last little worrying thought, but think positively: imagine all those beautiful and pleasant delights . . . remember . . . enjoy . . .

And if you still can't sleep, then accept the fact.

Get up, go to the lavatory, make a warm drink, have a little walk around the house — or even the garden — look up at the stars, gaze at the moon, wonder about the great mysteries.

Then go back to that warm bed, and start again.

9

Daily Life around the Home

There are all sorts of small precautions you can take to ease the difficulties of an arthritic hip in getting about the house. Invite your doctor and district nurse to come and have a look round, and you'll be surprised just how many suggestions they'll have to ease your life.

However, in general there are some obvious safety measures.

- Don't polish your floors, get rid of your small mats, watch out for curling corners and edges in the carpet, and repair any worn patches in the floor-covering, because if you slip and fall with an already damaged hip you may also get a broken thigh bone or fractured pelvis.
- Don't leave things lying on the floor, and be careful not to let the cat or dog get under your feet.
- Make sure that the treads of your stairs are non-slip, and a hand-rail on each side would help.
- Have good lighting, and take your time getting about.
- Remember that your hip-joint will move more easily and less painfully if you keep warm, so regulate the temperature of the rooms in which you spend most of your time. They don't have to be hot enough to grow tomatoes, but make sure you don't get too cold.

Now for making life easier.

- Don't pick up heavy objects, bags or suitcases, and certainly don't carry them very far. If you do have to pick up something heavy, keep your spine as straight and as upright as possible, so that your hips and knees do the bending rather than your back.
- When you make your bed, kneel on the floor rather than stoop to tuck in the bed-clothes. Better still, get a continental quilt.
- Go in for long-handled brushes and pans to avoid bending.
- Have a high chair or stool to sit on when doing the washing-up or the ironing.

Sitting comfortably

If you have a job getting in and out of an ordinary chair, raise the height of it on steady wooden blocks. But your feet must be able to rest firmly on the floor. Make sure that there are strong ends on the arm-rests to give you some solid support to press on when you get up or sit down.

Experiment with cushions or alter your position and angle to make yourself more comfortable, and take a small cushion if you travel by bus or train.

There are even special chairs with adjustable legs and raised seats, plus spring-loaded 'ejector' mechanisms which lower you from a nearly standing position or lift you when you get up — and some turn into full-length recliners. These do tend to be expensive, though what's money? I'd much prefer to spend what I have now on comfort and convenience than have it buried with me.

Remember that an ordinary chair with a hard seat and an upright back is better for you than a lounge recliner.

Other helpful hints and gadgets

Stairs

If you can't manage the stairs, even with hand-rails, because the steps are a bit too high for comfort, get a strong wooden box or block half the height of the step, make sure it fits the tread safely, fit a walking-stick to it for easy lifting, and go up or down half a full step at a time raising or lowering the box or block and placing it on the next tread. Slow, but sure.

Lavatory and bath

Using the lavatory can be both difficult and painful with a hip that doesn't allow you to squat properly, so fit a raised seat. They're not expensive, and they clip on and off — which means that other people can still use the one underneath. A handle on the wall will also be of great help in lowering yourself and getting up afterwards and two handles are even better.

Try to manage without such a seat if you possibly can, because excretion is more efficient the lower you squat.

Getting in and out of the bath can also be a tricky problem. The help of another person would obviously be a boon, and to be bathed with tender loving care is a pleasure in its own right.

A non-slip bathroom floor is essential, and a non-slip rubber mat on the bottom of the bath will give you an extra sense of security. Experiment with a low wooden box or even a couple of small steps to get in, and a strong board or seat across the bath will make getting down into the water that much more of a pleasure. And a couple of strategically placed handles on the bath and wall will give you added leverage.

Using a shower is also a good idea, either in its own cubicle or inside waterproof curtains at one end of the bath, with the unit attached to the taps. But do make sure of your footing.

Aids to getting around

Walking-sticks

To rely on any sort of assistance in getting about is not a weakness, but rather a sign of determination, so don't be too proud to use a walking-stick. Think of it in the same way as any other aid to getting around: you use a car as an aid to travel distances too far to walk, and you'd push your heavy luggage on a station trolley, and wouldn't you call a pair of good shoes an aid to walking? So why not use a stick?

Make sure that it has a solid rubber ferrule otherwise you may have it slipping away under you. Or why not go in for a tripod stick? It has three splayed feet on the end, will give a bit more security, and will stand up on its own if you have to let go of it for a moment.

Walking-frames

If your hip is badly affected you may have to consider a walking-frame which you use with both hands. It's usually made of aluminium tubing, has four sturdy legs, partly wraps around you like a protective railing, and you 'walk' it in front of you a short pace, and then catch up with one leg: another short pace with the frame, and you catch up with the other leg. It's as slow as climbing up the stairs, but very sure.

Some have a basket attached to the front so that you can do a

54

bit of shopping or change your books at the library, and some even have a flap which can turn down to become a seat if you get tired. What luxury!

Wheelchairs

It's unlikely that your doctor will allow your hip to deteriorate so badly that you'll need to use a wheelchair: you'll be put in for a hip joint replacement operation long before then.

But there may be special circumstances which will make it necessary for a while: perhaps a temporary acute stiffness or even an accident. In any event you'll be given plenty of good advice by both your doctor and those supplying it, but make sure that you all know precisely what you'll be using it for: indoors only, outdoors only, or both? Will you be pushed? or will you be propelling yourself? Does it need to be collapsible so that you can get it upstairs or into a car? And remember that detachable arms and hinged foot-rests will make it that much easier to get in and out of.

Driving

With thought and care it is still possible to go on driving a car with an arthritic hip, though, as with nearly everything else, take your time. So avoid motorways.

The driving itself is less of a problem than getting in and out of the car, but one simple idea is to pull back your seat when you get out. This will give you much more room to swing your legs round past the door and on to the kerb, and will make getting back in equally easy.

If you can afford it, there are specially designed swivel-seats which can be fitted, and these swing out from the car with you in them: all you have to do is stand up, and you're on the pavement.

If you can afford a new car, then you have fewer problems: choose one with a good height above the road, wide doors, plenty of leg-room, space behind the steering wheel, and a swivel-seat.

And experiment with various small cushions to make sure that you're sitting comfortably: there are even adjustable backrests.

Suitable clothing and footwear

With an arthritic hip you have got to ignore the dafter demands of 'fashion' and wear flat-heeled, comfortable shoes, which allow your feet plenty of room. To be able to walk without constriction is essential to keep your hip flexible. To totter around with cramped toes or high heels will only accelerate the deterioration of your damaged joint. 'Fashionable' or faulty shoes can cause deformed feet, strained leg muscles, and throw your hips and knees out of true alignment — which will cause uneven wear in your joints.

You may even have caused or at least contributed to your own damaged hip-joint by the shoes you've been wearing, so take professional advice from the trained staff at a good shoe-shop.

Walking barefoot is marvellous therapy, and you'll surely have healthier feet. Avoid hard pavements and roads, and try sandy beaches, meadows, lawns, paths of leaves through woodland . . . anywhere natural. There's even the appealing idea that to walk barefoot across grass which still has the morning dew on it will stimulate vital pressure points, improve your circulation, and give you an exhilarating sense of freedom and wellbeing.

In cold or damp weather warm clothing is essential for arthritics. Trousers will keep your thighs and legs warmer than even a long skirt, and men should wear long-johns rather than briefs.

There's not much evidence that cold and damp can actually cause arthritis, but they certainly make it feel worse. And a bleak day can lower even the highest spirits: things tend to look much more threatening when you're depressed. So wear bright colours. Grey woollen gloves and scarves are warm, yes, but yellow or crimson are more cheerful. And a fluffy rainbow hat will work wonders for your morale. There's even something rather comforting about the thought of red flannel underwear.

During cold weather your body uses more of its energy to keep warm. So watch the barometer: when pressure starts to fall, start to keep warm before the cold gets to you.

But on warm sunny days why not try sunbathing? There are plenty of secluded or naturist beaches, or even your own garden. The freedom and sense of innocent wellbeing will do you good, and so will the warmth of the sun.

10

Relationships and Dependence

Recognise when you need help

When you've got an arthritic hip you're going to be more dependent on others than you were before: immediate family, relations, friends, neighbours, your employer, colleagues or mates at work. You'll perhaps need help using the lavatory or having a bath, getting up and down stairs or on and off the bus, doing house work, out shopping.

You may have to spend so much time and spiritual energy on coping with your hip that you might be unaware of the effect you're having on those around you. You may be feeling low, but you can still try to smile a bit of a smile. Do what you can to help yourself, but when the going gets rough, admit it — and allow others to help you.

It's a question of balance: too little help and sympathy, and you'll suffer unnecessary pain, but too much fussy help and misplaced sympathy, and you'll be allowing others to do for you what you could do for yourself, probably lose the will to go on trying, and thus become totally dependent. Those around you will encourage and help — but you're the one with arthritis, and they can't overcome that *for* you.

It's your hip, and nobody else can walk on it.

Everybody you live or work with must be told that you've got an arthritic hip. There's no need to moan, but simply let them know that you're not quite the fit and healthy person you used to be, and that you'll be glad of their help from time to time.

Don't forget to let your employer know all about it: there might be a more suitable or less strenuous job available, or perhaps you could arrange a day off now and again, or shorter hours. You'll probably be surprised at just how many people are willing to lend a hand or a sympathetic ear.

Help from the hospital or clinic

Remember that other patients you meet in the doctor's waiting-room, or at the clinic or hospital, have all got a story to tell. It will be of great help and encouragement to hear how they have managed.

Indeed, some clinics and hospitals organize counselling sessions during which arthritics can tell each other about their problems, and it's both moving and chastening to meet other sufferers worse off than you and discover how well they're doing.

Be emotionally honest

Don't try to do too much, don't ever get too tired, always keep something in reserve, maintain a sensible balance between healthy activity and natural rest, get enough sound sleep. All that is the standard good advice. But you must also be able to say No as easily as Yes. Which means that as an arthritic you've got to be emotionally honest with yourself, stop agreeing when you disagree, don't do what you *truly* don't want to do and, if you have problems in getting on with other people, have the courage to face them.

You don't have to be destructive, don't have to barge into fragile situations with your great big fighting-boots laced on. It may be your husband or wife, your best friend, or your employer, or even *you* who's causing the problem. But, whoever and whenever, clear the air, release the tensions with love and gentleness.

Why not enjoy a stress-free life?

Put your fears into words

Put into actual words your conscious fears and other strong feelings.

We usually do this by complaining to our family or friends about other things, or we have arguments or quarrels, or we seek advice with little intention of taking it — anything as an easy way of avoiding the real problems.

But once you start telling yourself and others how you truly feel, it will get easier and easier to face your own truth. Don't merely *think* the words, *say* them, *hear* them, get them out into the open. And the words will defuse the suppressed emotions,

58

and release locked-away feelings you didn't know you had — not all of them destructive.

Avoid bad vibrations

Avoid what are known these days as 'bad vibrations', because the truth is that some people and situations can be damaging to you and your hip. Aggressive, complaining, nagging, irritable, or manipulative people can leave you drained or guilty, tensed or gloomy — and one-sided relationships are corrosive.

Who needs any of it? And who needs noise or dirt or horror or terror or violence or pornography? So why listen to that sort of music? Why read the books or watch the films or leave the television on? Why accept other people's nightmares?

Take responsibility for every situation: choose whether or not you want to stay in it. Don't ask how you *should* be responding, but how you actually *feel*: trust *your* feelings more than other people's opinions.

Keep active

Keeping active socially has obvious benefits, emotional as well as physical. Go on visiting friends, invite them back, exchange all your news, play Scrabble or cards or chess . . . do everything to keep up your interests in life, anything to keep out of your troubles.

And don't ever be embarrassed at your stiff leg and limp: other people will notice much less than you imagine.

You're not an invalid, don't give in, but come to working terms with what's happened. Otherwise your resentment may fuel the inflammation of your arthritis.

You're not a mere victim, but somebody who's beavering away hard at recovery. And to disguise your symptoms under a 'brave' face may make them worse: experience them to the full, and you'll reduce them to their proper size.

PART II

The Operation and After

11

The Hip Replacement Operation

*With gratitude to the late
John Charnley, surgeon*

About a year or so after the diagnosis of arthritis my hip was obviously the worse for wear.

I'd followed all of my own advice, tried to live as normal a life as possible, but those sudden bolts of pain were now becoming increasingly frequent and more persistent, and I was limping badly. I wasn't sleeping well, either, and was finding it more and more difficult to work. So my wife insisted on another visit to our doctor.

'Yes,' he said after a session of painful flexings, 'it's high time I put you in for the operation. I'll get you an appointment with the consultant.'

Arranging the operation

A month later I was examined by the consultant, who listened to my description of the symptoms, flexed my hip in several ever more painful ways, studied the latest X-ray, and then said: 'Why don't we think about putting in a new hip-joint?'

He then described what was involved: diseased bone cut away, metal ball cemented into the top of the femur, plastic socket let into the pelvis. It all seemed simple enough. If I were a private patient it could be done the following Tuesday.

'I can't afford that sort of money,' I said. 'It's on the National Health or nothing.'

'There's rather a long waiting-list,' he said, obviously concerned. 'I'm afraid I'll have to ask you to see me again in six months.'

'Six months?' muttered the voices of Job's comforters. 'You'll be lucky to get it done in under six years!'

And I was regaled with harrowing stories of how the whole National Health Service was running down, of gross mismanagement and neglect, over-worked doctors and nurses, ward closures . . .

National Health Service or private?

You may be faced by such a choice.

If, despite all the various drugs and treatments, you start finding it difficult to manage, and provided that you're otherwise healthy enough, you'll probably be recommended for surgery, so what do you do?

Wait on the National Heath waiting-list for as long as eighteen months or two years in some areas? Or consider having the operation done privately which, with hospital fees, will now cost two or three thousand pounds?

If you've got the money, don't hesitate. What's money when it comes to freedom from pain and stiffness? Or if you're in one of the private medical insurance schemes you'll have little difficulty, though do read the small print.

Or perhaps you could raise the money on a bank loan or by taking out a second mortgage, though remember that it will be several months before you'll be back working and earning again.

Or, like me, you'll have to wait, in which case get your name on that waiting-list as soon as possible. Don't just think or hope your name *is* on it: make *sure*.

And please don't feel bitter about the apparent unfairness of money being able to buy the privilege of health: this is the way of the world in which we live, and to brood about it won't do your aching hip any good.

For where is it written that life has to be fair?

Surviving the waiting period

Kindly friends rallied round: 'Folk Medicine,' they said. 'Nature's Way.'

And, with a total lack of conviction, I drank enough cider vinegar to pickle a small elephant, blackened my teeth and tongue with blackstrap molasses, scattered wheat-germ on my oatmeal porridge, wore a copper bangle on my left wrist. I even considered carrying a dried potato in my trousers-pocket.

'What about the Devil's Claw?' they said.

I had a chilling vision of the Black Mass.

'The *what*?'

'The Devil's Claw,' they said. It turned out to be some sort of herb-root tea made from a wicked-looking plant found only in the Kalahari Desert of Namibia.

But I survived.

Then, six months later, a letter came which arranged the next appointment with the consultant: August, bright August.

'Yes,' he said after a brief but excruciating flexion of my left leg, 'Fairly rapid deterioration. Have to have you in as soon as possible.'

'When?' I said, hardly daring to hope.

'At the end of September, or the beginning of October.'

The relief was indescribable.

The preliminaries

He then asked me a lot of questions, and your surgeon will also probably want to know more about you and your circumstances. You might think that some of the required information is perhaps a bit irrelevant — but you'll soon see what's wanted: a fuller understanding of you as a whole person.

Questions about your general health are obviously essential: How's your heart? Blood pressure? What about indigestion? Are you over-weight? A smoker? Ever had a major operation?

Other questions will be on your way of life: Are your married? With children? Have you recently been divorced or bereaved? Or do you live alone? Do you need to climb stairs? What about your work? Will you be able to manage for the weeks and months after the operation? And so on . . . with some of your answers perhaps revealing problems and stresses that could interfere with your recovery.

You'll probably have to be over fifty, as the materials of the artificial joint have to last as long as you do. You'll have to be seriously inconvenienced by your arthritic hip: that is, your ability to earn your living and the quality of your life must be badly affected.

Your whole physical condition will be checked and tested

several times before the operation, because the more the surgeon and the hospital staff know about you, the more successful they'll be. Everything possible will be explained to you: the procedures, its benefits, and the risks involved, and the more *you* know about what's going to happen, the better the outcome.

Going into hospital

What will actually happen to you in hospital depends almost entirely on the surgical and medical procedures followed by your particular surgeon and the nursing staff, but perhaps my own experiences will be an indication of what you can expect.

Monday morning, early October, and I had all the usual uncertainties, the prideful reluctance at now having to be dependent on others . . . fear of the unknown.

But, from the first smile of the secretary who greeted my wife and me to the cheerful welcome of the sister on the male surgical ward, I knew I was among friends. There was an air of human warmth and assurance and unflustered efficiency.

My wife stayed to help me settle and get into bed, we said our goodbyes until the evening . . . and even the bed was comfortable.

Yes, all would be well.

Preparing for the operation

I had two blissful days being prepared for the operation: reading and looking out of the window at the autumnal trees, more than adequate food, visits from my wife.

I had a further X-ray: 'Just to make sure they know what they're looking for in there,' said the radiographer.

I was exercised by a physiotherapist: 'Essential that we keep these thigh and leg muscles in good nick,' she said. 'Especially when you're up and about again.'

I was examined yet again by doctors: pulse, heart, respiration, reflexes, muscle tone.

I had a special visit from the anaesthetist: 'I like to have a look at the customers,' he said.

I was shaved by an orderly . . . belly, genitals, hips, thighs:

'Keep yourself powdered after it's all over,' he said, 'it can get a bit irritating as it grows.'

I had several baths laced with antiseptic, and the site of the operation was marked.

They even showed me the *prosthesis*, (Greek for a thing placed or inserted, an addition to the body of an artificial part) the sort of ball-and-socket joint which would be replacing my own rather war-weary one.

'It has to be carefully selected for each case,' they said, 'with each of you a different size and shape. Hence all these X- rays. We have to know the precise dimensions needed.'

It was strange to be holding the two pieces in my hands, the metal ball and shaft surprisingly heavy, the plastic socket light, the fit smooth, perfect.

'Demonstration model,' they said. 'You should see the real thing.'

There was another visit from my wife on Tuesday evening, all the inadequate words said, yet all the love expressed.

I could have nothing to eat or drink from midnight.

Then there was another antiseptic bath on Wednesday morning.

A first injection: 'This will only make you a bit sleepy,' said the nurse, 'and your mouth will start going dry. You can clean your teeth, but try not to swallow any water.'

About the rest of that day I remember very little: the dry mouth, gentle drowsiness, being wheeled down the long corridor to the operating theatre, a few mumbled words with the orderly . . . swinging doors . . . the anaesthetist in a green gown . . . lights . . . shining . . . then that swirling black cloud of merciful oblivion.

The operation

The operation will be performed by a specially competent and experienced surgeon, and requires extra facilities and equipment not available in every hospital. The technical name for it is *arthroplasty*, which is the Greek for joint-moulding, with *plasty* sharing the same root as plaster and plastic. So it means what it says: moulding or repairing a joint.

The hip-joint is thickly surrounded by layers of powerful muscles. The ball is on the top end of the thigh, which is the largest and strongest bone in the body, and the socket is deeply seated in the pelvis, being simple, sturdy, and well protected. The work requires a major operation lasting two or three hours under a general anaesthetic.

It's a miracle of bio-engineering, surely one of the most impressive advances of modern surgery, which, with contemporary methods of anaesthesia and the use of antibiotics to prevent or control post-surgical infection, has become remarkably safe.

We owe a deep debt of gratitude to the late John Charnley, the British surgeon who, with his colleagues, developed the technique at a hospital in Lancashire after the Second World War. He was an internationally recognized specialist in orthopaedic surgery, and he and his team devised not only the operational procedures but also the various parts of the artificial joint: a highly polished cup made of polyethylene plastic to replace the damaged socket in the pelvis, and an equally highly polished ball on the end of a long tapering stem to fit snugly into the shaft of the thigh bone. This combined ball-and-shaft is usually made from a stainless cobalt-chromium-molybdenum alloy, which, with the plastic, is resistant to wear and essentially inert in the body, and thus almost eliminates the danger of tissue reaction. The shaft is cemented into the reamed-out top of the thigh-bone with methyl methacrylate. All of these materials are being improved all the time, and the resulting joint is probably stronger than the original hip.

The procedure consists of removing the whole worn ball and the top inch or so of the thigh-bone, reaming it out to take the stem of the new ball, cementing it into place, then fitting the new plastic socket into the pelvis, and finally making the necessary adjustments for a good fit.

The results are almost miraculous . . . at least to anybody who has had an arthritic hip-joint for a few years.

After the operation

I came round in a gentle confusion of quiet voices, reassuring faces looking down at me, driftings of sleep, movements of darkness on darkness, gradual awareness of peace and warmth . . . *and an absence of pain in my left hip and leg.*

The next day I was stiff, on my back, had a wedge-shaped pillow between my knees to keep my legs at the correct angle for healing, and a sandbag propped against the outside of my left ankle.

'Now remember,' said the nurse, 'no matter how much you want to, you mustn't try to turn over on your side.'

There was a plastic drip-tube feeding into my right forearm, a pair of similar tubes draining blood and gunge away from the surgical wound — but I felt fine. Though all I wanted to do was turn over on my side!

However, there were compensations: I cleared a full plate for lunch, and my wife came in, smiling, as close to tears of love as I was.

Yes, I was back in the real world again.

12

Walking on Two Hips Again

Your recovery depends largely on you: your inner reserves and resources, your attitude of mind, your sense of humour, and how well you co-operate with the various treatments, but obviously, a lot also depends on the particular post-operational procedures of the surgeon and the hospital staff.

However, all being well, you can expect to be out of bed and on your feet three or four days afterwards, and walking on a frame or crutches within a fortnight or three weeks.

'When you can get in and out of bed by yourself,' said one surgeon, 'on and off the toilet, in and out of a chair, and manage a flight of stairs, you're ready to go home.'

If you work at it, you can be walking without crutches in a month of six weeks — though, again, this rather depends on your age and general health.

Indeed, recovery is as important as the operation, and you'll be fully prepared, given all manner of good advice and suggestions for coping with the stresses and physical difficulties of the next few months. My own experiences were, I hope, typical.

Early physiotherapy

The day after the operation, I was being exercised on the bed by the physiotherapist: 'Thighs, legs, and toes,' she said. 'It's essential that we keep you mobile, maintain muscle tone, circulation. Nothing too strenuous. Flexions to start with, toe wrigglings.'

Ten minutes, and my legs were trembling.

'That's the ticket,' she said. 'See you tomorrow morning.'

In a few more days I was able to visit the lavatory at the end of the ward, trundling along on a wheelchair, which was a triumph.

I had several blanket-baths, the warm water a blessing, the towels a comfort, with that lovely sense of being looked after, and clean again.

I had another X-ray to see how things were progressing, and early the next week I was trundling down to the physiotherapy department, and being taught to take my first few tentative steps in a walking frame.

Exercises, exercises . . .

Exercises are a major part of rehabilitation, and here are some I was given.

- Stand up, hold onto something firm for support, the back of a chair — or even the sink.
- Keep back upright, swing affected leg forward and back. Repeat, standing on affected leg.
- Swing affected leg to side. Repeat, standing on affected leg.
- Keep back upright, bring knee up towards chest as far as you can. Repeat with other leg.
- Hold on to your support with both hands, and slowly squat several times trying to get down slightly lower each time.
- Sit on the edge of a table or bed with a rolled towel beneath your knees for comfort. Hang a small bag of sugar or flour or dried beans on your left foot, starting with about two pounds, then straighten your leg, bending it up at the knee. Repeat several times . . . and then do the same for your other leg.
- Gradually increase the number of repeats each day . . . and feel it all doing you good.

Making progress

Next out come the stitches, leaving a thin neat scar about nine or ten inches long down the top of your thigh above the joint.

You can now have your first proper bath. Bliss!

Then you can attempt the first flight of stairs, one heaving step at a time, hanging on to the hand-rails, with coming down more nerve-racking than going up.

By the end of the second week you're an expert.

Then comes the first walk outside, fresh air, all that sunshine, through the hospital grounds as far as the main gates and back.

And so on, always a little more, a little further . . . two sticks . . . one stick . . . and then you're walking unaided!

71

At home

When you get home treat yourself rather like a new car: run-in your hip-joint slowly, don't go too fast at first, and certainly not too far.

One more important point: All the time you are recovering, you are entitled to all manner of State benefits, either as weekly allowances or services such as Home Help. Your doctor will be able to advise you, and the staff at your local office of the Department of Health and Social Security will be more than helpful.

But remember that these benefits are yours *by right*, and if you have any difficulty obtaining them, go to your nearest Citizens Advice Bureau.

What else?

Now start living life to the full again!

PART III

Alternative Therapies

13

Do We Need Conventional Medicine?

My operation was a complete and unqualified success: I no longer had any pain in my left hip, could walk, climb the cliffs, swim, saw and chop wood, dig the garden, but a few years afterwards I started to get those old familiar twinges in my other hip . . . and the twinges became jabs.

This time I needed no persuading by my wife to go to the doctor.

'Well,' he said after the obligatory session of symptoms and flexings. 'It can only really be the one thing, can't it? There *were* indications in your last X-ray.'

And we agreed that all the walking about on a painful left hip had thrown most of my weight on my right one, which had started to wear.

'You know the story,' he said, and made out the familiar prescription for one hundred analgesic tablets.

In two or three years I could have the operation.

Why could so little be done? What point or purpose was there in going through all that again? *Could* orthodox medicine possibly be wrong?

Orthodox medicine

Until quite recently it was reasonable to believe that medical science had all known diseases on the run: the great killer epidemics no longer killed, new cures for everything else were being pushed on to the market faster than they could be advertised, and we stood at the painless frontiers of a Brave New World.

Yet, today, the ancient scourges seem to have been replaced by newer ones: cancer, heart conditions, arthritis. And medical science, for all its vaunted research, can't yet do much about them: still can't cure the common cold, still can't manage more for a headache than suppress it with drugs, still chases after miracles . . . with tragic results. You only have to remember Thalidomide.

Doctors don't *always* know what's best for us.

Why are we beginning to doubt?

Part of the reason is that in orthodox medicine, as in so many other scientific studies, an almost mechanistic view of cause-and-effect has long since supplanted the more traditional 'spiritual' explanations of why we fall ill.

'If it can't be measured,' said the cool researchers in their white lab-coats, 'it doesn't exist.'

But, as many people are now beginning to understand, the scientific theories upon which modern medicine has been built are quite simply fallacious. Disease isn't *only* caused by pathogens: all manner of other factors are involved. As Brian Inglis writes:

'It is as if our personalities dictate the type of disorders we are most likely to suffer from, our lifestyles decide the level of risk or vulnerability, and stress precipitates the outcome — the disease.'

Orthodox medicine was once sure of its answers, but even some doctors are now doubtful that it was asking the right sort of questions. It's becoming obvious that there's more to the body than its functioning as a machine, that not all effects have simple causes, and that some of the standard remedies and procedures do as much secondary harm as primary good.

Another factor in this erosion of the old faith in orthodox medicine is that these days there are too few doctors for too many patients, and that most of them just haven't got enough time to go into all your human details. You're the tenth or twentieth person they've seen that morning, the waiting-room is still probably full, and they've got a busy day in front of them.

Little wonder that, even with the best will in the practice, it's easier for them to scrawl prescriptions for indigestion or lack of sleep than to listen to your personal troubles. They mean well, but the road to disease is papered with those easy prescriptions.

It's also true that the medical establishment remains largely wary of unorthodox wisdom, has occasionally ignored or actively condemned ideas that have later proved to be correct and curative, and yet has often been wrong about some of its own recommended treatments.

Once upon a time the almost universal 'cure' for every known disease was blood-letting — either by knife and basin, or leeches from the nearest pond.

More recently the prime cause of many diseases was thought to be constipation: 'All those poisons clogging the body — clear 'em out!' Strong emetics and purges and frequent enemas were the favoured methods.

And, even more recently, patients with arthritic hips were immobilized in bed, sometimes for weeks at a time, with sandbags stacked around their legs to prevent any movement . . . or even set in a plaster-cast from waist to knees.

These days it's drugs for nearly everything, with more drugs to counteract any side-effects.

What does all this mean for anybody with an arthritic hip who doesn't fancy batches of analgesic tablets every four hours even when necessary? Who could do without being a burden on family and friends? Who doesn't want to drag around for two or three years merely waiting for the operation?

I'm not knocking analgesics, nor my own hip-joint replacement, merely pointing out the possibility of there being another way, other therapies.

Other therapies

The clue to the nature of other therapies is that most doctors tend to talk about the 'management' of arthritis, rather than its treatment or cure: and that much of this 'management' has to be done by you — for though there are many drugs currently being prescribed, a lot depends on your own attitude towards the effects of the disease.

Some people obviously have a stronger need or will to believe than others, and are 'healed' or gain relief from all manner of procedures which can't possibly 'work' in any strictly 'scientific' way: a copper bangle on the wrist, a dried potato in the pocket, hands lain on in prayer. Have faith, and you can 'remove mountains' . . . or cure an arthritic hip-joint.

And even the most orthodox of medical researchers have to admit this element of faith, because in the standard clinical tests for any new drug the patients are given either the active drug itself, or an inert and harmless tablet called a *placebo*. This is a Latin word from the Roman Catholic liturgy for the dead, meaning 'I shall please' — which is also used sardonically by doctors to describe a prescription given merely to satisfy a bothersome patient.

And it's an established fact that the results for the placebo in clinical trials are often better than those for the drug being tested . . . indicating that as much probably depends on the faith or optimism of the patient as on the drug.

Applying alternative therapies to osteoarthritis

Today some of the old ways and therapies involving faith and self-knowledge are being rediscovered.

Many doctors still regard them as a mess of superstition, ignorance, and credulity. 'If it's *miracles* you're after . . .' they say.

But I must speak as I have found.

Of all these alternative therapies currently available I have only considered those which claim to have an effect on osteo-arthritis.

Orthodox medicine alleges that the treatment of osteoarthritis is a 'fertile field for speculation and superstition', but this is probably because its own field remains largely barren.

True, it can be admitted that the causes of the disease are vague or uncertain, and that some patients are apparently healed without any proper treatment.

In my case, the proof of the treatment is in the hip-joint.

My left one was healed by the surgeon — for which I will never cease to be grateful . . . but my right one is being healed *without* the knife.

More and more people are now trying these alternative therapies, the major attraction of which is that their practitioners are as much concerned for the whole person as they are with the alleviation of symptoms. For to treat only the symptoms is to neglect their causes: it's not the *disease* that needs the help, but the *person* .

Now it must be freely conceded that there have been all manner of curious 'remedies' for osteoarthritis: zinc or brass heel-plates screwed on one or both of your shoes, various coins or Holy Medals held by sticking-plaster to different parts of your affected leg, copper bangles or a dried potato, various herbal teas, a diet of cherries or grapes or grapefruit . . . and Christiaan Barnard mentions one he was told about: blood from a baby's umbilical cord, centrifuged to obtain the plasma, which is administered by injection. 'Shakespeare would have liked that,' he adds.

However, it's unfortunately true that there are many completely unqualified people milking a fat living from the exploitation of pain and distress: quacks, frauds, more than one 'guru' from the Mysterious East with your money in mind — even well-meaning but self-deluded enthusiasts.

Given that arthritis tends to come and go, and that you'll feel better on some days than on others, it's inevitable that sometimes the use of a dubious 'remedy' will coincide with an improvement — when it will get the credit, and the huckster will get your money.

And, again, just like doctors, not all of even the qualified therapists are as well qualified as others — and you might get lumbered with a dud.

None of which is any judgement on a genuine therapy.

Testing the therapist

So please don't be too starry-eyed about these therapies: some of them have never been adequately tested, and you mustn't believe everything you're told. Find out for yourself, retain your critical intelligence.

There are two very rough and ready tests you can use: one of the therapist, and the other of yourself.

It has been suggested that if any of these alternative therapies suddenly became acceptable to orthodox medicine it might lose much of its attraction, not just for its patients but for its practitioners. Because some therapists do take a perverse pride in the opposition they get from the orthodox, almost as though the opposition itself is a guarantee of correctness or seal of approval.

'If the British Medical Association condemns us, well then, we must be right!'

But your health is much too important to be risked on a

therapy which might be based on resentment — so, in choosing a therapist, watch out for too much knocking of orthodox medicine.

Testing yourself

The second rough and ready test is of yourself: Are *you* a suitable case for treatment?

Some of the ideas and attitudes involved may be so unusual, so beyond your fringe of acceptance, that you might find them hard to take seriously, and while a sense of humour is always essential, you must be serious enough to give them chance to succeed. In other words, you must have faith — and how can you have faith in anything you regard as ridiculous?

Again some of the ideas may outrage your own sense of your self and how you function, may question your motives and assumptions, may even embarrass you.

For example, one theory which is basic to several therapies is that some sufferers from osteoarthritis tend to be emotionally restricted and inflexible in their views: you perhaps have rigid joints because you have a rigid mind . . . the harder your heart the stiffer your body, the colder your soul the worse your pain.

Such a suggestion may leave you spluttering with anger, but might it just be true? Because your anger could well be the first symptom the therapist would want to examine as an indication of the probable cause of your condition. If you reject the very idea out of hand, the therapist can hardly help — let alone cure.

Most of us have romantic illusions about what life 'ought' to be like, and often cling to impossibly high ideals . . . which can result in repressed resentment and even anger directed towards other people. With the help of a therapist start to accept yourself, admit the truth of your own feelings, face your resentments and anger . . . and you may start to loosen the rigidity of your arthritic hip-joint.

But you can't if you resent the concept of anger as a cause.

However, from my own experience I can assure you that the relief of self-knowledge will be therapeutic.

Having had a 'strict' upbringing, I had always been ashamed about nakedness, and associated it with sexual guilt, but I am now an unconcerned naturist who enjoys both my own and the equally innocent nakedness of other people. I can't *prove* that it has helped directly with my arthritic hip-joints, but I'm now certainly less rigid in body as well as mind.

So there it is. If any of these ideas outrage you, if human nakedness is a sin in your book, if the thought of vegetarianism is funny, then it's unlikely that you'd be fully responsive to the principles of natural health which are the foundation of these alternative therapies. You *must* be open to new and perhaps disturbing influences.

The principles of natural health

So, briefly, what are these principles of natural health we'll be considering?

- That most of the diseases we suffer from have come about as the direct result of our way of life and what we eat and drink.
- That there's usually a connection between the sort of person you are and your disease or illness.
- That it is of little use concentrating on symptoms while neglecting their deeper causes.
- That to find out why you are ill is as important as finding a remedy, for self-awareness and understanding are the first ingredients of any medicine, the first steps in any treatment.

On these terms, an illness or disease is your body trying to tell you something. For example, a heart-attack may be saying that you must slow down, restore the balance between being and doing, because the heart is more than a mechanical pump, but also the symbolic centre where you ought to be feeling more and deeper emotions.

Any illness or disease may be a similar warning that you need to pay attention to how you are living, what you are living for — even why you are living at all.

And the days or weeks or months during which you are ill may be the very time you need for rest, thought, mental and spiritual refreshment, and the creation of a whole new way of being and doing. Your body may be both warning *and* giving you the opportunity to change.

So why not find out what *your* arthritic hip-joint is trying to tell you?

14

Alternative Medicine

To try one of these alternative therapies requires a change in your attitude towards your own health. You are now going to accept full responsibility for yourself, start making more of your own decisions, learn about diet and exercise and how to cope with stress.

Mind you, don't buy the plausible notion that *all* diseases are always our fault, that we are fully responsible for everything that happens to us — otherwise you're back with the old nightmare of disease being the result of some sin or other. Sometimes, yes: if you smoke you must be prepared to risk lung-cancer, or if you are sexually promiscuous you mustn't be surprised if you contract a venereal disease.

On the other hand, you may have lived what you believed was a healthy life, and yet *still* have an arthritic hip-joint.

The purpose of these therapies is to find out what you lack for a more abundant life.

What is holistic health?

John Rowland, a consultant herbalist, has most elegantly expressed the fundamental idea upon which they work: 'to create a condition, by means of any therapy that can make a contribution, whereby the healing powers of the body can be aroused.' And he mentions fasting, diet, vitamins and minerals, hydrotherapy, herbal medicine, the use of aromatic oils, deep breathing, exercise, homeopathy, acupuncture, osteopathy, physiotherapy, and several other such related means and methods.

It's called *holistic health*, from the Greek word *holo*, meaning whole . . . with the further rich complex of associated meanings: to be in one piece, integrated, holy, or hale, to be free from defect or disease, to be healthy. So the therapist doesn't treat diseases or parts of the body, but considers your *whole* body in order to make it hale and healthy again: *where* you live is as important as *how* you live, and *why* you've got an arthritic hip may be the answer as to what to do about it.

Your therapist will try to bring relief to your body, but will also include your mind, your emotions, your feelings, and your soul or spirit. Because your attitudes to your world, your feelings about yourself and other people, what you eat and drink and how you breathe, the places where you live and work, the company you keep, the things you do and the thoughts you think — all these have an effect on your health, and to ignore them is to be less than whole.

Many doctors still depend on drugs rather than regard the patient as a person who needs to be made whole, whereas the alternative therapists are more interested in *you* as a *person* than in your symptoms. The first one I ever went to was a perfect example: I told her that I'd had the replacement operation, and that now the other hip-joint was deteriorating. 'Yes,' she said, 'but how are *you*?'

That's the holistic approach.

Therapists have (or make) the time to regard you as a unique human-being, worth their respect and complete attention. They value you for *who* you are, not necessarily *what* you think yourself to be. They point out that disease is only partly caused by pathogens, but is also the result of an imbalance among a variety of social, personal, and economic factors.

Because you are unique, their treatments take into account your character and circumstances. Further, they demonstrate that good health is not merely the absence of disease, but a state of vitality and positive well being: inner harmony, personal fulfilment, enthusiasm, confidence, optimism . . .

'We must learn to live at peace with ourselves and with each other,' they say, 'and to live in harmony with the world which sustains our lives.'

You have a personal responsibility for maintaining your own health, then, and the key to this sort of guided self-healing is the sincere desire to rid yourself of suffering. You must now become an active partner with your therapist, not remain a body on which the treatment is performed. And this personal reponsibility is more difficult than swallowing aspirin or even staying on the strictest of diets.

Deep-rooted troubles or ingrained habits are probably causing your arthritic hip-joint — so you have to be prepared to find out what they are, and then to *do* something. The success of these therapies largely depends on what you bring to them.

In fact, the major difference between the orthodox and the alternative approach is that many doctors are still reluctant to admit anything so damaging to their self-image, whereas the therapists make healing use of your essential co-operation.

First, a warning

By all means trust in the self-healing powers of your own body. But if you don't respond to these natural treatments, please don't hesitate to make use of the full resources of contemporary orthodox medicine and surgery. For both orthodox and alternative medicine share the common aim: healing the sick.

In fact, you could get your doctor's approval of the therapy you intend to try: it's not essential but the holistic approach is one that willingly embraces all possible help, and your doctor is uniquely qualified to monitor your progress.

Besides, it's not only good sense but good manners.

At the frontiers of orthodoxy

Even within the bounds of orthodox medicine there are several treatments which, though they haven't gained much general support from the profession, have still been effective with some cases.

For example, various doctors in America are using large doses of radiation to destroy certain blood cells which they believe are responsible for some forms of arthritis, and it has been reported in the medical press that the pain and swelling can be relieved.

However, radiation is undoubtedly dangerous, and it may be years before the long-term results are known.

Dr William Fox and the diphtheroid organism

In this country, Dr William Fox has worked for over fifty years as a general practitioner and specialist in the treatment of arthritis and rheumatism, and one of his original ideas is that arthritis starts as a low-grade viral infection, which, if diagnosed early

84

enough, can be successfully treated with an injection of diph-theroid preparation.

As you probably know, some germs cause disease, but others are necessary to life: for example, there are organisms teeming in your bowels without which you'd die. The body's immune system, part of our natural defence against infection, is always ready to deal with attacks by bacteria trying to use us as a place to feed and breed. When any of these harmful organisms enter a wound, armies of white blood cells gather to engulf and destroy them. And the usual vaccine is prepared by breeding a particular strain of these harmful organisms in the laboratory, and render-ing them inert — and thus harmless. This culture is then given to you in a small dose, mostly by injection, thus stimulating your body's normal healthy defence against such organisms, so that when the real ones attack your system you're in a much stronger condition to resist.

Dr Fox had noted that most arthritic patients lacked the diphtheroid organism, which is not a disease-causing germ, and he conceived the idea that perhaps these patients were suffering because this harmless organism had been driven out and replaced by some of the harmful ones. He tested this by trying the effects of an injection prepared from two strains of diph-theroid, in the hope that it introduced into the body something which might be beneficial. Many other doctors have suggested that arthritis is caused by an infection, and that a vaccine should be developed. The results were astonishing — an improvement rate of ninety-two per cent — and he's been using this treatment ever since, for over thirty years, with not a single case of adverse reaction.

Unfortunately, he has been met with the almost traditional negative response from the majority of his colleagues. Re-member Lister and his long struggle to introduce antiseptics? How hard the 'experts' fought against chloroform? Sir Herbert Barker and bone-setting?

However, your doctor ought to know about this method of treatment, as it has been fully reported in the medical literature, so please ask if the idea attracts you.

Christiaan Barnard and the green-lipped mussel
An extract of the green-lipped mussel, *Perna canaliculus*, a

species found along the shores of New Zealand, is claimed to be an effective supplement or possible alternative to orthodox therapy in the treatment of both rheumatoid and osteoarthritis. Some doctors have reported that it reduces the amount of pain and stiffness, improves the patient's ability to cope with life, and apparently enhances general health.

It certainly helped Christiaan Barnard, who has chronic rheumatoid arthritis, and he was still using it in 1985, so it's well worth asking your doctor about.

Amino acids

There's evidence to suggest that some amino acids, such as histidine, seem to be missing from the blood of many arthritics. Amino acids are essential to the health of the body: most of them are produced by the body itself — but many must be provided in the food you eat.

We are all different, and have differing nutritional needs, but we would all probably benefit by eating those foods in which the necessary amino acids are plentiful: eggs, milk, liver, fish, soy beans, brown rice, peanuts, peas and beans — with sufficient fresh fruit and vegetables to supply the vitamins.

They're excellent foods, anyway, so your health will improve whether or not there's any improvement in your arthritic hip.

Enzymes

There is also good evidence to suggest that some forms of arthritis may be caused by enzymes leaking from the cells lining the joint, and that these break down the cartilage and destroy the synovial fluid like acid.

Enzyme is Greek for leavened, the idea being that these complex organic substances act rather like yeast in the fermentation of dough: transforming other compounds in a sort of soluble ferment without actually themselves changing, destroying without being destroyed.

The main supportive protein of tendons, bones, cartilage, and connective tissues, is *collagen*, a word based on the Greek *kolla*, meaning glue. It's the breakdown of this collagen which causes the main damage of osteoarthritis: high quality collagen depends on the presence of ascorbic acid, or vitamin C which has a chemical action on some of the amino acids which are the forms of protein used in its production by the body, so if the collagen is deprived of vitamin C it either produces a poor quality replacement or no replacement at all. And the cartilage begins to wear away. Thus, a good supply of this essential vitamin will obviously help to slow down or even halt the damage.

In fact, it's been demonstrated that vitamin C and vitamin K3 actually seal the walls of the cells lining the joint, prevent leakage of enzymes, and the condition of the whole area improves.

In scurvy, for example, a disease caused by a lack of vitamin C, easily cured by the addition of fresh oranges, lemons, or limes to the diet, the victims could hardly walk or endure the pain of their damaged joints. So may not arthritis also in part be caused by the absence of vitamin C from our diet?

To supply any deficiency a well-balanced diet high in protein is usually recommended, along with plenty of fresh fruit and leafy green vegetables. One of the other advantages of vitamin C is that the body absorbs only the amount necessary for its needs, and rapidly excretes any surplus, so you can happily make sure of meeting those needs by drinking lots of blackcurrant-juice or taking supplementary vitamin C tablets.

Enzymes and lead

It has also been suggested that one of the enzymes responsible for the breakdown of the cartilage of a joint and the destruction of the synovial fluid is activated by lead. So exposure to lead may have started the deterioration of your hip-joint, and it's obviously worth investigating.

Lead poisoning is caused by handling or working with it (especially if you don't follow the statutory safety precautions), flaking lead based paint, drinking water from lead pipes, eating too much tinned food (when the contents of the tin are contaminated by the soldering of the joins), but largely by the heavy car-exhaust pollution of the air from the addition of tetraethyl-lead to petrol. For example, vegetables grown alongside motorways have been found to contain fifty times more lead than is considered tolerable in manufactured foods, and people living near any area of congested traffic usually have astonishingly high levels of lead in their bodies.

87

If you have been exposed to any of these sources, then do tell your doctor — it may well be *your* specific cause.

Calcium is a powerful agent against lead, and renders it almost non-toxic in the body, so drink plenty of milk, and eat cheese and natural yoghurt. And hard water, which contains more calcium than soft, is better for your hip-joint.

15

Nature Cures and Nutritional Therapies

The principle of nature cures

The general principle of a nature cure is exactly what's implied: nature will cure if given the chance.

Most of us no longer live close to nature, but unnaturally: in cities rather than small communities, eating too many junk foods, drinking too much alcohol, watching too much television, not getting enough sleep, wearing too many clothes, not getting enough fresh air — living under stress rather than in peace and happiness.

We have lost touch with our instincts, we hardly ever see the sun rising or setting, the moon is merely a potential space-station, and we mark the wheeling of the stars in their courses by checking our horoscopes. And as for the passing of the seasons — isn't it merely briefs in summer and long-johns in winter? Cards and presents at Christmas and chocolate eggs at Easter.

Those who believe in the cure offered by nature recommend that we must start to rediscover what our bodies are trying to tell us, eat fresher and better food, stop smoking, drink less alcohol, enjoy more fresh air and free sunshine, get more exercise, be more gentle, more loving, more at one with the world in which we all live.

If that lot sounds a bit too much, then few of the nature cures are really for you.

Pass on, friends.

Naturopathy

The best-known of these cures is naturopathy. This is based on the idea that disease is caused by your body trying to get rid of the accumulated wastes which have been steadily piling up in your body through years of wrong habits, and the whole treatment consists of expelling these, and then developing better habits of living and eating.

We can obviously make ourselves ill by eating the wrong foods — 'wrong' in this case not only means contaminated foods which make us vomit or feel sick, usually within hours, but also polluted, adulterated, or denatured foods that may take years to inflict their long-term damage on us.

A naturopath will relieve the pain of your hip by completely natural means, and will encourage your own self-healing by suggesting a fast or perhaps a colonic irrigation, which is flushing out your colon with warm water. And then you'll help your vitality by various diets. No drugs are used, but hydrotherapy, mud-packs, massage, herbal remedies, vitamin and mineral supplements, and courses of exercise.

So first you get rid of the pollutants and toxins, and then you provide the best possible nourishment to help your body deal with the arthritis in the most natural way.

You start with a fast: depending on the advice of your therapist, you go without food for one or two days, and drink only water or fruit juice.

An easy way to fast for twenty-four hours is to miss your evening meal on the first day, and breakfast and lunch on the second. The fast is then spread over a couple of days, and no complete day is spent without any food at all. This fast is intended to detoxify your body, and get rid of its accumulated poisons.

We usually do this by excretion, urination, sweating, and breathing — though, occasionally, when we've eaten something really bad for us, we vomit it up from the stomach. When these natural processes no longer work properly, we're in trouble, and most of us would benefit from such a digestive rest once or twice a month.

Some naturopaths recommend an enema or colonic irrigation at the end of this fast, just to make sure that your body is thoroughly purified and in natural working order again. *Enema* is the Greek for 'send in,' and it's merely a 'sending in' or injection of warm water to give your rectum and lower colon an internal bath. It's not necessarily a 'fun' experience, though it doesn't have to be unpleasant either.

You then continue by eating nothing but fresh ripe grapes and melon for two or three days, about a quarter-pound of each for breakfast, lunch and evening meal. You have nothing much to drink, as there's enough fluid in the fruit. Don't worry if you have to urinate more than usual, as this flushing out of your whole system will be entirely beneficial.

For the next week or so you drink apple or grape juice, and eat meals of apples, pears, grapes, peaches, raw salads, and cottage cheese. You can also have natural yoghurt, a little molasses, and the occasional drink (hot or cold) of vegetable yeast extract.

You then stay on a more or less strict diet, again depending on your therapist's judgement of your needs: mostly vegetarian, and certainly avoiding refined white sugar, white bread, cakes, sweets, tea, coffee, alcohol, and all tinned and chemically preserved foods. (About such preserved foods there's the phrase: 'If it doesn't ever rot, don't ever eat it.' There must be something suspect about cakes and biscuits that last for a year without apparently going bad.) Some therapists however allow a little lean meat, chicken, and fresh fish.

After a month or so, when your body has recovered from years of neglect or abuse, and you're probably feeling better and healthier than you've been since you were a child, you gradually enlarge the choice of foods. But, again, a lot depends on your therapist. However, you'll almost certainly avoid the 'foodless foods' of our time, and be required to eat everything fresh and pure, organically grown and free from chemicals.

But, whatever you do, don't get neurotic about it. Better to laugh on fish-and-chips and pickled onions than look grim as you count the calories in a grated carrot. Simply give your body all the proper nourishment it needs, help it to get rid of everything it doesn't want, improve your heart and circulation by getting enough exercise, breathe deeply, walk on the sunny side of life, smile, love — and you're taking the nature cure.

The nutritional therapies

Nutritional therapy is based on the idea that a cure for osteoarthritis is less likely to be found in the laboratory than in the kitchen, less in drugs than in foods.

Eat well, which *doesn't* mean seven-course banquets, and you'll be healthier than if you eat badly. Which is not to say that those who eat well are never ill, but simply that unsuitable food doesn't help an arthritic hip.

It seems reasonable to assume that what we eat and drink must have some effect upon our health: our bodies are biochemical machines fuelled by our food intake. So the wrong fuel could obviously cause trouble in the works, as is undoubtedly true with diseases of the heart. How healthy do you think you'd be if you lived largely on hamburgers, sweet pickles, chips and crisps, chocolate cream cakes, and strong tea?

However, the United States Arthritis Foundation denies that any form of arthritis is either caused by food or the wrong combination of foods. Eating 'special foods or eliminating others from your diet will not cure arthritis'. But it does agree that if you're 'poorly nourished' you won't be as healthy as you could be, and that this in turn 'will affect your general health and your ability to resist or endure the physical wear and tear of arthritis'. This opinion is shared by the British Arthritis and Rheumatism Council: 'In general,' they write 'the medical profession does not feel that diet plays a great part in the treatment of these diseases.'

Some doctors are scathing about even the possibility of there being a diet that will improve your arthritic hip. Others, equally well qualified, disagree, and have demonstrated that the adoption of a diet of natural foods can bring effective relief to arthritis and eliminate the need for pain-killing drugs.

Though they all agree that people with an arthritic hip ought not to carry too much extra weight around, and 'weight control through diet' is the standard recommendation.

Again, gout is a well-known form of arthritis, and sufferers are almost always advised to avoid all foods high in uric acid: fatty foods, liver, kidney, hearts, offal generally, meat extracts, game, thick gravies, fish roes, herrings, sprats, sardines, anchovies, whitebait, salmon, caviar, asparagus, spinach, strawberries, rhubarb, and to cut down on all protein-rich food. In addition, they must also avoid carbonated drinks, heavy beer, sparkling wines, strong red wine, port, and many other kinds of alcohol.

So if these foods cause arthritic gout, how can anyone be dogmatic enough to deny that these same or other foods may also have similar effects in other forms of arthritis? If not eating them will relieve gout, then why not other comparable conditions?

And there are now many doctors who accept that we are what we eat, and that some foods are better than others for your hip joint.

Dr Collin Dong's diet

Dr Collin Dong, for example, the well-known American specialist, was afflicted with arthritis that 'no amount of pain-killers and anti-inflammatory drugs seemed to help', and yet he cured himself by means of what is still regarded by the orthodox as a 'highly contentious' diet. It's radical enough by any judgement, and difficult to follow if you're devoted to the processed foods of our time — but he claims that it's 'tantamount to a cure'.

Briefly, you eat all sorts of fish, all fresh vegetables, vegetable oils, margarine free of milk solids, egg whites, honey, nuts, soya-bean products, rice, wholemeal bread, onions and garlic, any kind of flour, and a little sugar, but you *never* eat any sort of meat except (occasionally) breast of chicken, fruit of any sort (including tomatoes), any milk or butter or cheese or yoghurt or egg yolks, vinegar, pepper, chocolate, dry roasted nuts, alcohol, and any food to which any chemical flavourings and colourings and preservatives have been added — especially monosodium glutamate. You *can* drink tea and coffee.

He first presented this 'recipe for a longer, happier, and pain-free life' in 1974, and since then thousands of sufferers from arthritis have found it effective. His book is called *New Hope for the Arthritic*, and it's published by Granada.

Dr Jarvis' diet

Dr Jarvis of Vermont, an equally famous practitioner, recommends two teaspoonsful of cider vinegar and two of honey in a glass of water, sipped during every meal.

Honey, of course, has long been regarded as the perfect food, contains no harmful chemicals, and has very little waste. The flavour when modified by the vinegar is often hard to enjoy — yet it grows on you.

At every breakfast you take one kelp tablet, made from the various brown seaweeds and containing 'at least sixty minerals or trace elements, more than twelve vitamins, and twenty-one amino acids — all in perfect balance.' And three times a week you add one drop of iodine to the honey and vinegar at one of your meals. All of these products can be bought at any health-food shop.

You also avoid wheat breads and cakes, wheat cereals, white sugar, citrus fruits and their juices, and muscle meats like beef, lamb, and pork.

And thousands of people have reported great success with this diet, which, at the very least, can't do much harm. If it works for *you* then accept the gift with gratitude.

Arthritis and Folk Medicine, by D.C. Jarvis, is published by Pan Books.

Dr Giraud Campbell's diet

Dr Giraud Campbell, another American specialist, offers the 'easing of swelling in your joint within a week', the 'relief or often the complete elimination of pain in two weeks or less', 'more natural movement' in the vast majority of cases in three weeks or less, the 'restoration of damaged bone structure in three to six months'.

But you have to be willing to give up tea, coffee, soft drinks, alcohol, bread and all other flour products, canned and all other processed or manufactured products, icecream, sweets, and live on organically grown raw fresh vegetables and fruit. As with naturopathy, you begin with a fast, and work up to the complete diet in a month or so, gradually adding fresh dairy milk, natural cheese, free-range eggs, fresh fish, and lean meats.

There's much more to it, which you will have to find out from the book or with the help of a therapist, but, if it ends your pain and improves your hip, who cares whether or not it meets with the formal approval of orthodox medicine?

A Doctor's Proven New Home Cure for Arthritis, by Giraud Campbell is published by Thorsons.

Other diets

There are now literally dozens of similar diets available, and probably hundreds of thousands of sufferers have benefited from them. It's obvious that they differ widely, often contradicting each other in a confusion of prohibitions and recommendations, and I am simply not competent to determine if there's any direct connexion between the diets and the benefits, or if it's mostly a matter of faith.

People vary, and what works for some may not work for all. But it doesn't really matter *which* of them might work for you, nor even *why* any of them work at all . . . only that they bring relief to some.

Unfortunately, there are few general agreements about what we should eat and drink for good health.

'All you need,' state the accepted authorities, 'are regular balanced meals drawn from a wide range of easily available foods.'

Who could argue with such bland advice?

The only trouble is that fresh healthy foods are no longer so 'easily available'.

Almost every packaged or tinned or frozen product you buy in the High Street is stale, devitalized, with most of its natural goodness destroyed, artificially flavoured and coloured, 'enriched' by the addition of synthetic imitations of the very essentials previously refined out of it, and then embalmed in preservatives.

'Fresh' vegetables are probably a week or more old, months if they've been imported: they have probably been grown in a sort of chemically saturated sponge rather than organic soil, and sprayed and drenched with dangerous weedkillers and insecticides.

A notorious experiment has demonstrated that rats fed on a famous breakfast-cereal did less well then rats fed on the chopped cardboard of the boxes in which the cereal was packed.

And then we wonder why we feel 'run down' and why we suffer from arthritis!

As a rule don't ever eat food that doesn't appeal to your own tastes: to force yourself will do more harm than good. But if it has been recommended by a therapist you trust, at least give it a chance by trying to make it appetizing.

Suppose you've been advised to eat raw cabbage, and you can't stand cabbage raw *or* cooked.

Well, grate it finely, mix with sliced onion, dress in olive oil and lemon juice, with chopped fresh herbs as a garnish. Arrange on a plate with three different sorts of cheese and a scattering of assorted nuts and enjoy yourself.

There's never any need for simple food to be served unattractively: there are even easy ways of making last night's leftover mashed potatoes into a delicious breakfast.

Two other suggestions.

Eat five of six small meals a day rather than three large ones, as this gives your digestion the freedom and continuity to work without the strain of too much bulk all at once. Chew your food well, and thus swallow it in a better prepared condition for the stomach to deal with it.

To eat healthily isn't self-restraint, but self-realisation, and can be a daily exploration into new pleasures of taste and texture: it must never be mortification of the flesh, but rather an unalloyed blessing to it.

With the possible relief of your arthritic hip the greatest blessing of them all.

Allergies

Another theory worth considering is that your osteoarthritis may be the result of an allergy — a now familiar idea. The word is based on the Greek *allo*, other, plus *ergon*, work, together meaning 'something which works in another way'.

For example, Charlie can eat oysters, and they 'work' by making him feel good . . . but Mary might break out in a virulent rash if she so much as sat at the same table. On *her* the oysters 'work' in another way: she's allergic to them.

We know about hay-fever. Certain people are affected by the airborne pollen from plants and trees, which causes severe irritation of the mucous membranes of their eyes, nose, and throat. *We* can sniff the gentle breeze, and enjoy the smells of the countryside . . . *they* will sneeze and weep and feel ill.

Other people get headaches if they eat strawberries or tomatoes, others are allergic to detergent and so on.

Very few orthodox specialists in osteoarthritis acknowledge that it may be caused by an allergic reaction to certain foods and even environmental pollution. But there are now so many cases that it's difficult to understand how they can go on denying the truth of their own medical literature.

Patricia Byrivers has written a most optimistic book about her own experiences.

She developed arthritis 'while still at school,' and, 'after twenty years of misery and an increasing reliance on cortisone', she finally discovered that her symptoms were due to the foods she was eating practically every day.

She had no knowledge that arthritis could be allergy-based, and it took her 'several years to determine the various guilty foods'. In her book she describes how the 'process can be shortened to an initial week'.

Goodbye to Arthritis, by Patricia Byrivers, is published by Century-Hutchinson.

Treating allergic arthritis

There are now several flourishing clinics in this country which offer allergy detection and treatment, not only for osteoarthritis, but migraine, asthma, and may other mysterious complaints for which orthodox medicine hasn't yet much to offer.

You'll have to answer all the usual questions about any previous illnesses, your symptoms, and your present diet and the allergist will make quite sure that you really have got arthritis, and not one of the more serious bone-corroding diseases.

Then you will have a restful week or so on a 'low-risk' diet of bland foods which, in the opinion and experience of your allergist, only rarely act as allergens (or 'triggers') in cases of arthritis. At the end of this time your pain will almost certainly have eased, and you'll probably feel better than you have for months or even years. Initially, to be truthful, some people actually feel slightly worse: tired or aching . . . but that's merely the body getting used to living without the foods which may have been causing the trouble, rather like the 'withdrawal' symptoms you go through when you first stop smoking.

To this basic diet will gradually be added various other foods until your particular allergen has been established. It could well be one of your favourite foods, and the choice is then yours: that food or your arthritic hip.

All this testing can be done with you as a full-time patient in one of these clinics, which tend to be expensive places, or you can attend for a number of consultations and follow the diet at home — in which case you'll need to be extremely strict with yourself, because even so much as one nibble or sip of a forbidden food can interfere with the whole process.

You could try it out for yourself: all you have to do is learn which foods bring on the pain. Keep a food and pain diary for a few weeks: note what you have to eat and drink for every meal, and also note when your pain gets worse, and then see if there's any connexion between what you ate yesterday and what you're suffering today. If fish on Fridays is followed by pain on Saturdays, then stop eating fish. Easy as that.

But do please tell your doctor what you're doing, because the whole process can take a long time without skilled advice.

One suggestion which might give you a running start: It's been established that many arthritics have a sweet tooth, with years of stirring refined white sugar into tea, too many toffees, too many soft drinks . . . so why not check your own intake?

16

Homeopathy

What is homeopathy?

When we become ill we mostly believe that our symptoms are the result of an attack by one or other of the pathogens, some germ or virus or poison: that some harmful organism is responsible.

Homeopathy, the theory of Samuel Hahnemann, an early nineteenth century German biochemist, is based on the assumption that your symptoms are really the results of your body trying to resist the attack. 'Far from seeking a way to suppress symptoms,' he wrote, 'it may be desirable to take some form of treatment calculated to help the resistance.'

The word itself is derived from the Greek *homoios*, like, plus *pathos*, suffering, together meaning a likeness of feeling: the technical definition of homeopathy being 'that theory which regards disease as being curable by remedies which produce in a healthy person effects similar to the symptoms of the disease to be cured'.

Homeopathic treatments

Behind this idea is the general holistic principle that we all possess a vital motivating force integrating our body, mind, and soul, that can correct any 'aberration from the normal state of good health'. Homeopathic treatments are intended to work at this deep level of power, with the added advantage that, because only unhealthy cells or tissues respond to them, there can be very few dangerous side-effects.

The orthodox doctor would prescribe a drug that lowers temperature for a feverish patient, but the homeopath would prescribe one to raise the temperature, because fever is the body's way of fighting off the disease — fighting like with like.

This is by no means an unusual medical procedure, as the whole orthodox theory of immunization is founded on it: small doses of smallpox are used to protect you against the real thing.

But Hahnemann lost the approval of the orthodox (not to

stress that of the drug companies) by then developing the apparently ridiculous procedure of reducing the strength of the drugs he used to almost impossible dilutions.

The drugs themselves were standard, produced from herbs and minerals that have been prescribed for centuries to treat illness. But Hahnemann discovered that 'high doses of medication tend to intensify symptoms', where 'small doses tend to strengthen the body's natural defences', that it's not quantity that works, but quality: potency wasn't related to strength.

If he 'diluted the medication to one part in a hundred of distilled water', and 'successed' it (rapidly shook the bottle until 'infusion was complete'), the 'remedy actually became *more* effective'. And he went on diluting until, 'on accepted scientific principles there will not be so much as a molecule of the original drug left'.

(To non-enthusiasts, this process can be likened to emptying a small cup of cold tea into a large lake, stirring well, and taking three drops of the mixture as a remedy for terminal cancer.)

Yet Hahnemann claimed the 'remedy would be more effective the greater the dilution' — a paradox that still baffles most doctors.

And this remains the radical difference between orthodox medicine and homeopathy: currently standard treatment with drugs involves high doses, with the almost inevitable side-effects, while the homeopath dilutes the substances in successed distilled water and alcohol to make a tincture, sometimes to only one part in a billion, thus avoiding all possibility of any unwanted reactions.

Sceptical doctors still demand to know how such minute amounts of active substance can possibly have any appreciable therapeutic effects?

Some clinical trials on homeopathic remedies have shown positive results, while others have shown no significant difference between one homeopathic remedy for arthritis and an inert placebo. These results give little support to those homeopaths who prescribe for osteoarthritis. Though, with some justification, the homeopaths dispute these findings, and claim that their remedies are more effective in the treatment of arthritis cases than conventional medicine, with these same controlled trials 'proving that they were right'. And even the cautious *Lancet* has given 'qualified approval' to their case in this dispute.

Christiaan Barnard considers it 'interesting' as an effective remedy for arthritis, but goes on to suggest that 'so far the merits are not proven'.

One fact *is* certain: it can't possibly do you any harm.

Most homeopaths would undertake to treat osteoarthritis of the hip — but, obviously, if your joint is already badly damaged you can't really expect immediate results.

Make sure that you consult a properly qualified practitioner, preferably one who is also a qualified doctor: then you will get the best of both disciplines.

The flower remedies

These were discovered by Dr Edward Bach at the beginning of the century, and they form a graduate branch of homeopathy.

He qualified as a bacteriologist in London shortly before the First World War, became a brilliant practitioner, contributed several major clinical techniques to orthodox research but then grew dissatisfied, studied to qualify as a homeopath — and eventually made the discovery which gave his name to the theory at the symbolic root of the Bach Flower Remedies.

'Patients who respond to various orthodox remedies,' he wrote, 'do not necessarily share the same physical symptoms,' but 'do share the same mental and emotional state'. And he believed that 'disease is in essence the result of conflict between soul and mind — so long as our souls and personalities are in harmony all is joy and peace, happiness and health'.

This seems reasonable enough. If you are in harmony with your true self and your world you will be happy and healthy. Do wrong to yourself or to others, and you're in conflict, ill at ease . . . ill or dis-eased.

So Dr Bach didn't prescribe his remedies for any physical complaint, and none of them is a specific treatment for osteo-arthritis. But they are claimed to deal with 'causative factors', and are 'recommended for people with underlying emotional problems which may be found to relate to physical symptoms'.

And he proposed a number of emotional characteristics and the problems associated with them, symbolically matched.

- For example, pride and rigidity leads to stiffness of the body.
- Hate leads to loneliness, violent temper, and hysteria.
- Selfishness leads to neurosis and neurasthenia.
- And deliberate ignorance, the refusal to see or hear the truth, leads to poor vision and deafness.

If, with the help of a therapist, you begin to understand yourself as 'resentful and bitter', or 'dominating, inflexible, ruthless, intolerant, arrogant, and critical', then you have in you the 'negative emotional problems' which are often found in sufferers from osteoarthritis.

Hard to admit, perhaps. Yet, in the words of Carl Jung: 'People will do anything in order to avoid facing their own souls.'

But even to consider the possibility that those around you see these qualities in *you* will be therapeutic, the beginning of self-knowledge, which will perhaps lead to humility, a much more flexible approach to life, tolerance, acceptance of others.

And what might all that do for your aching hip?

Using flower remedies

The remedies are simple, being the 'essences' of 'benign wildflowers', which 'grow above ground in air and sunlight'.

Edward Bach would gather them in the early morning when the dew was still heavy upon their petals, choose only perfect specimens, and distil their essence in one of two ways: either boiling then gently in pure water and then filtering, or steeping in pure cold water for three hours under the full sun.

Anybody can do this, and he always insisted that his remedies could be prepared and used by those who needed them: they are 'absolutely benign in their action' and could 'never produce an unpleasant reaction under any conditions'.

If the simplicity and symbolic 'rightness' of the idea attracts you, why not discuss it with the Bach therapist? There's a Bach Centre at Mount Vernon, Sotwell, Oxfordshire, OX10 QP2, from which you can get books and free advice.

Herbal remedies

'Nobody who has ever experienced the soothing effect of a dock leaf on a nettle sting', states the advertisement in a natural health magazine, 'can doubt the efficacy of herbal remedies'.

Many doctors are merely dismissive: 'There is no evidence to suggest that they are worth buying.'

But herbalism isn't new: in ancient Egypt, China and India it was one of the major sciences, and knowledge of the healing powers of plants has been accumulated over thousands of years. And, after all, most modern synthesized drugs began as preparations from them. For example, the original source of aspirin was the willow bark which contains the natural salicylic acid currently synthesized in the laboratory.

It's interesting to remember just how close the ancient and modern still are in the drugs industry: Thomas Beecham, founder of the pharmaceutical and proprietary conglomerate, and Jesse Boot, who started the famous chain of chemist shops, both began as herbalists and their descendants, though they made their millions in other ways, still have a soft spot for some of the traditional remedies — though they're given 'scientific' descriptions these days.

Natural herbs are certainly milder in action, and have many fewer side-effects.

Principles of herbal therapy

'Today', writes Tony Hampson, a well-known consultant herbalist, 'the medical establishment seems to take the view that a medicine only works when you know why it works. And yet herbal medicines have had the longest clinical trial in history.'

Many plants produce various substances as a defence against being attacked by insects or being eaten by animals: and through long experience some of these substances have been shown to be of great healing use in the treatment of human ailments.

The orthodox procedure is to isolate these substances, define their specific action on the body, and then synthesize them in the laboratory, to be administered as 'wonder' or 'miracle' drugs, and, very often, another drug has then to be devised to treat the side-effects.

Tony Hampson states that 'practitioners of natural medicine accept that it is the *whole* plant in harmony which provides the remedy, not just the active principle. This element of harmony is part of the philosophy of holistic medicine.' So the herbalist uses the whole plant in the preparation of treatments in the belief that the 'secondary plant products are better administered to the body in the correct balance put there by nature.'

Unfortunately, as Brian Inglis has dryly observed, 'the range of agreement among herbalists over what remedies to use for particular disorders is surprisingly small.'

To use herbs as a specific remedy to remove symptoms is to do no more than to use synthetic drugs, and I very much doubt if any herb could do anything very much for an arthritic hip joint. But herbs are an essential contribution to a healthy way of life, and most herbalists regard their remedies as part of the holistic health movement. So by all means relieve the pain of your hip with a recommended herbal treatment, but remember that if you can see it as part of your larger attempt to remove the deeper causes you'll be more likely to succeed.

If you've been advised to give up tea and coffee, there are several perfectly adequate herbal substitutes to be had from any health food store, with several either soothing or stimulating flavours, and you make them in the same way as tea or coffee.

And do please try a herbal bath sometimes: they come in sachets: mixtures of various dried herbs, which you steep in the water. There are some lovely and sleep-inducing perfumes, and you simply wallow happily for as long as the warmth lasts, and then go to bed smelling of high summer and wildflowers.

To find a herbalist, ask around in health food stores, read the natural health magazines, study the articles and advertisements. Make sure that you aren't going to be fleeced by anybody unscrupulous and that your therapist is a qualified member of either the Faculty of Herbal Medicine or the National Institute of Medical Herbalists.

17

Osteopathy and Other Techniques

As the two Greek words suggest, *osteo*, bone, and *pathos*, suffering, this is the treatment of suffering bones: a system based on the theory that diseases can be remedied by the direct manipulation of the bones and (indirectly) of muscles, blood vessels, and nerves.

It is 'concerned with the establishment and maintenance of the normal structural integrity of the body'. Bodily structure and functions are completely inter-dependent: if the structure is altered in any way, then the functions alter. Alter functions, and the structure alters.

In the case of osteoarthritis, these alterations are caused by poor posture and the wear-and-tear of daily life, which together bring about 'mechanical disturbances', especially in the pelvis and spine.

So, theoretically, and often in fact, it is possible to restore a wearing hip joint to its proper position, and realign the surrounding muscles and tendons to maintain it there — the sooner the better.

Do tell your doctor that you're intending to consult an osteopath: they are now medically 'respectable' after many years in the orthodox wilderness, and your doctor will probably be able to recommend one.

The treatment

The osteopath will take your general case history, but will also watch how you walk into the room, how you stand and sit, and will be looking for connexions between the information you provide and how you hold yourself. In addition (and this should come as no surprise) you will be watched for any signs of emotional stress.

Then the osteopath will examine your whole body, and move each joint through its range of motion, and the subsequent session of treatment will involve your arms and legs being used as levers for manipulating full mobility and restoring them and your spine to their normal positions, thereby relieving abnormal tensions in muscles and ligaments.

But remember that it's not really an on-going form of treatment for osteoarthritis of the hip joint, but First Aid for neglected bones — corrective, rather than curative.

The sheer relief after a session can be overwhelming.

Yoga

Some teachers of yoga claim that certain of its *asanas* or poses, with their associated meditations, can have a beneficial and healing effect on arthritis of the lower back and hips. These *asanas* are mostly spine-stretching and hip-bending, which improve the posture, tone the thigh muscles, increase the blood supply to the whole region, and relieve the stiffness and pain.

Yehudi Menuhin, who has practised Yoga for many years, talks of the 'tragic spectacle of warped people working out their own imbalance and frustration on others', and recommends it as a way of restoring a 'primary sense of measure and proportion' and preventing physical and mental illness.

If yoga can do anything for either your own peace of mind or the suppleness of your body, it's at least worth a few experimental sessions. There are teachers and groups all over the country, and most adult education centres run day or evening courses.

The Alexander Technique

This therapy is designed to first treat, and then prevent, a variety of diseases and disorders by an apparently simple system of 'postural changes'.

It was discovered by Frederick Matthias Alexander, an Australian actor who worked on himself for many years to rectify the inexplicable loss of his voice during performances. The solution to his own problem seemed astonishingly trivial: he was pulling his head backwards and downwards and sucking in his breath whenever he began to speak. He taught himself to stop doing this, and had no more trouble with his voice.

But he subsequently established a direct relationship between these seemingly trivial 'uses' of the body and many much more serious complaints than the occasional loss of the voice. Indeed, Professor Nikolaas Tinbergen, winner of the Nobel Prize for Medicine in 1973, affirmed the possibility that 'stress-related ailments could benefit from the Alexander Technique, including various forms of arthritis'.

It's much more than a simple correction of the posture, but is concerned with the proper use of the *whole* body. We must be completely aware of our body and how it functions, and be willing to change the bad habits of a lifetime.

However, it can't really be self-taught, and requires the time and personal attention of a qualified practitioner to correct your posture and movements. But the whole idea is still based on Alexander's observation that the action which most often precedes wasteful or harmful movements is a slight contraction which pulls the head backwards and down. This compresses the spine: repeated hundreds of times a day over a span of many years, it interferes with the smooth operation of the muscular and nervous system and all the vital organs.

And this is only *one* destructive habit, the first of a whole series that will follow if it occurs unchallenged . . . which can lead to round the clock tension and chronic muscle and joint pains. So we need to prevent the neck from contracting unnecessarily by using our conscious mind to change our subconscious muscle patterns. And the essence of the whole process is to begin any movement by moving your head in the direction you are going and away from your body, and then letting your torso lengthen by following in that direction.

It's obviously much more complicated than that, and you have to learn all over again to stand and sit and walk with the natural grace of a young child, consciously learn to be unselfconscious.

Your doctor should know about the Alexander Techniques, and may even be able to recommend a practitioner, but, as always, please make sure that he or she is qualified.

Rolfing

Related to the Alexander Technique is Rolfing, a form of

'structural processing' named after its developer, Ida Rolfe. It uses deep massage to realign the body to its proper posture, which is then 'structurally balanced', with the body vertical and in harmony with gravity.

When your body is out of alignment you are bent over by gravity, and your body can't function correctly: hence, perhaps, your damaged hip joint. And an 'unbalanced' body is unstable, and demands tremendous muscular strength and energy to keep it from toppling.

It's also claimed for Rolfing that the strenuous massage involved is often accompanied by a great emotional and energetic release and purge of unresolved tensions: sadness, fear, joy, rage, anger. Because it's not just a simple matter of restoring physical equilibrium, but of understanding how feelings create postural change. To rebalance the physical body will often lead to personal growth.

Hypnotherapy

Another Greek word *hypnos*, sleep . . . meaning to 'serve or to treat by or through sleep.'

But hypnosis, unfortunately, is still often thought of as being either sinister or merely entertaining: a melodramatic villain putting the 'fluence' on some sweet innocent maiden, or a stage hypnotist making some weak-willed dupe believe that a floor-mop is Marilyn Monroe.

However, it has a long history, especially for treating pain, and is becoming increasingly respectable. So, if your osteoarthritis is in any way linked to excessive emotional stress, hypnosis would bring about a suspension of your conscious mind, and enable the deeper levels to become accessible to the powers of suggestion. Hypnotherapy, therefore, is a procedure for placing helpful suggestions in your unconscious mind, which may then work on your various mental and bodily systems.

It doesn't claim to heal or cure directly, but simply to cause reactions which may ultimately lead to relief of the condition. And it's now often used to help with smoking, over-eating, and even major surgery. So at least its power over pain need not be questioned.

True, successful hypnosis depends on total trust and relaxation, so if you've got any serious reservations it won't work: you can't be hypnotized against your will, though it is reassuring to know that you can't possibly do anything in the deepest trances that you wouldn't do when awake.

Uses of hypnotherapy

Hypnotherapy, then, is most effective in dealing with conditions in which there's an 'emotional overlay', when your emotional or psychological state is considered to be largely the cause of your 'dis-order', the well-known psychosomatic factor, where a disease of your *soma*, or body, is caused by something wrong with your *psyche*, or soul.

You must have faith in the process, trust in the therapist, must be willing and receptive, otherwise you'll both be wasting your time. It's as if you hand over responsibility for your actions to the therapist, relaxing completely under sensitive guidance, and then the therapist uses this freely given permission to enable you to understand yourself, and thus bring about your own healing.

In a calm and relaxing atmosphere, you'll sit in an easy chair or low down on a comfortable couch, breathe in and out deeply, and then the therapist will use a gently reassuring voice to 'talk' you into a trance, slowly, persuasively.

When you are relaxed, and your mind is free, the therapist will then begin to use direct suggestion that your symptoms are going to be relieved, or will explore with probing questions if or why any psychological problems could be affecting your arthritic hip, and thus facilitate whatever form of treatment is to be used.

In general, the main purpose of hypnotherapy is to assist relaxation and lessen tension, which will give increased confidence and ability to handle problems. Your symptoms won't go away directly, but you'll be less tense and stressful, and many people with osteoarthritis have reported reduced pain and improved mobility.

Hypnotherapy is now medically 'respectable', and more and more doctors are qualifying as hypnotherapists, so your own doctor will almost certainly be able to help you one way or the other, either by recommendation or actual therapy.

Therapies based on energy flow

Acupuncture

This is currently the most famous of these alternative therapies, and its name is based on two Latin words: *acus*, needle, and *punctus*, to puncture or prick, meaning to prick with a needle.

An early and once common orthodox 'cure' for arthritis was plunging a needle into the affected part, but this sort of rough and ready treatment has obviously got very little to do with the much more subtle Chinese procedure.

When information about it first became known in the West it was derided by the orthodox, who called it lunacy and worse, but it is now beginning to be accepted — mostly because the evidence for its success is too overwhelming to be denied. Tens of millions of television viewers have now watched major operations being performed with acupuncture as the only analgesia. About a fifth of all operations in China are performed with its help, and it is slowly being accepted as a genuine adjunct to standard medicine.

True, some doctors remain sceptical: 'Time does the healing, 'they say, 'and acupuncture gets the credit.' And it has even been suggested that the filmed operations were staged for the cameras, and the 'patients' were actors trained not to show pain.

What acupuncture does. The idea behind acupuncture is that the body has a complicated network of interlocking meridians all over it. These carry your various vital energies to where they are needed, and when you are ill or 'not yourself' the meridians become sluggish and out of balance. So by stimulating them at certain specific points, either by pressure or by the insertion of needles, your body's essential flow and balance of forces may be restored.

Qualified acupuncturists insist that it's not simply a matter of correct diagnosis and accurate positioning of needles, with you as a passive spectator, but that you must co-operate to the full: they 'tune up' the system, but the motivation to use the corrected power has to come from you.

You'll have a very thorough examination before any treatment is suggested, with many questions about your attitudes and feelings.

110

The stainless-steel needles are extremely fine, with tiny heads, and you'll hardly feel them being inserted: some sensation, yes, but not pain — nothing like a hypodermic injection. So that's the least of your worries.

Results of acupuncture. Reported results for the procedure range from 'brilliant success' to 'total failure'. There is little evidence that it has any significant effect on the underlying inflammation of arthritis, or the progression of the disease, though there seems to be temporary relief of pain for some patients.

Dr Felix Mann, a pioneer in the use of acupuncture for arthritis, who has been working with it for nearly thirty years, is direct and honest: 'Osteoarthritis of the hip joint, except in rare instances, responds only temporarily.'

However, there are several clinics where it's being tested to see if it can help with chronic pain. So, if you have severe pain, which doesn't lessen no matter what's tried, then talk to your doctor about being put in touch with a qualified acupuncturist. After all, *you* may be one of the instances when it *will* have a significant effect. Obviously, don't expect too much. Try it by all means, for even the partial or temporary relief of pain *could* give you a breathing space.

Remember that acupuncturists treat people, not symptoms.

Shiatsu

This is the ancient Japanese art of acupressure, a form of therapy which uses finger pressure instead of needles. But the basic theory is similar: as long as the bioenergy flows smoothly through the meridians we experience well-being, but when this energy is 'blocked' it stagnates, and we experience negative emotions and ill-health.

The therapist uses almost the same interconnections along the meridians as in acupuncture, and these respond to various degrees of pressure from fingers and knuckles, which brings relief from pain, reduces fatigue, and stimulates the body's natural ability to heal itself.

Foot reflexology

This is closely related to both Shiatsu and acupuncture, being

111

based on the same principle that a life force or energy flows through the body along the meridians, except that it concentrates on the ten terminal points of these meridians in the toes and feet. One reason for this difference is that the feet are parts of the body with least depth to them which renders the meridians easier to reach and manipulate.

Using the thumbs and fingers, the therapist will massage and stimulate various of these terminals, restore the energy flow to its correct balance, and thus improve your general circulation and activate sluggish glands and organs to improve their function.

It's both stimulating and relaxing, and I can vouch that it dispels stress and eases pain. But only a qualified practitioner could possibly do it adequately, though even a loving massage of the feet will be pleasurable, quite apart from the good it will do for your general well-being and peace of mind.

Kinesiology

This is also closely related to these other therapies which work on the flow of energy along meridians, but the use of the Greek *kinesis*, movement, implies that it has more to do with the movement of muscles than with the stimulation of pressure points. Indeed, it's been called the 'science of muscle activation', and its purpose defined as the 'restoration of that muscle balance which is essential to good posture'.

Based on the theory that relative muscle strength and tone can be utilised to diagnose disease, its muscle-testing procedures are used to tap the innate intelligence of the body in order to assess the energy levels of the life forces which control it.

There's a relationship between the meridians, each muscle, and the corresponding groups of organs which share the meridians. By detecting imbalances in the muscle groups it is then possible to diagnose which organs are weak or diseased. And therapists claim that they can detect dietary deficiencies, allergies, organ dysfunctions, and the extent to which psychological factors are involved.

Applied kinesiology. Otherwise called 'touch for health', this is a method of treatment which includes adjustments to your diet, but mostly consists of the application of touch as a way of transmitting or arousing healing forces. The therapist will be skilled in the usual methods of massage, which in themselves are a powerful source of sensuous pleasure and well-being but there will also be the most delicate fingerings of your meridians and acupressure points, even caresses, which realign your energy flows and leave you revitalized.

The kinesiology therapist who helped me has done as much for my right hip as the surgeon did for my left. No, my osteoarthritis hasn't gone away yet . . . but it's going. Thank you, Rikki.

Water and heat

Water is used in various ways in these alternative therapies: as a drink, obviously, and in several sorts of washing and bathing.

Some therapists recommend the drinking of six or more pints of water a day as a method of flushing the system of poisons, and even that you should avoid ordinary tap-water — which, after all, is known to be a chemical cocktail of chlorine, fluoride, and whatever also is the latest fashion in additives. You can either buy bottled pure spring-water, which tends to be expensive, or use a filter. Any health food store will have bottles and filters.

You may also be given alternate hot and cold baths, or wrapped in wet sheets, showered, sprayed, steamed, or soaked in various herbs or salts.

On the theory that all life began and evolved in the oceans, and that the salts in your blood serum are closely linked to those in the sea, some therapists make great use of sea water in the treatment of osteoarthritis. And I have been greatly helped by swimming and playing in the sea.

Sweating to reduce pain

It's agreed by orthodox medical practitioners that profuse sweating can often reduce the pain of osteoarthritis and this can be brought about in a variety of comforting ways:

- You can be wrapped in several layers of warm blankets, with or without hot water bottles.
- You can be wrapped in a plastic sheet, and then in an electric blanket, with the therapist swathing your neck and head with

113

towels that have been dipped in iced water — essential to prevent over-heating of the brain and the body as a whole.
- Or you can sit in a steam-cabinet, and sweat for twenty or thirty minutes.

The pleasures of a sauna need little recommendation: a small room built of fragrant pine-wood, benches, hot stones; the dry heat induces the necessary sweating and cleanses the body of impurities, and then the steam when water is poured on the stones. You can massage yourself briskly with a rough towel to improve skin tone and circulation or even use birch twigs in true Finnish style.

Religious healing

Religious healing is obviously too profound a subject for any brief account to do it proper justice, but, in faith, you have everything to gain and little to lose by considering the possibility. Because both the religious and the healing task are essentially the same.

If you are a Christian the promise is that if you open your heart and mind to Christ, accept his love and forgiveness, then inner healing will result. And this inner healing has got a great deal to do with the bodily healing of osteoarthritis.

Avoid big public meetings where fervent evangelists claim to work instant miracles without any prior diagnosis, and go to an accredited healer who will take time to pray and meditate with you. Your local priest or pastor ought to be involved from the start, 'for let everything be done decently, and in good order'.

18

Working Rules for Osteoarthritics

- The Golden Rule about osteoarthritis is that there *are* no golden rules.
- Freedom from pain isn't the only liberty: work for freedom from arthritis.
- Liberty means responsibility: do you really want either? If so, you must change.
- Who can, does. Who cannot, suffers.
- Take care to get what you need, or you will be obliged to put up with what you get.
- Assume a greater responsibility for your own health.
- Stop believing that doctor always knows best: sometimes, yes, perhaps even more often than not, but never always.
- The answer to your damaged hip-joint may well be drugs and an eventual operation – but perhaps you're asking the wrong questions.

    There is a lot of research into causes and cures going on all over the world: tissue rejection, genetics, the possibilities of a vaccine, the control of inflammation by means of a specific protein rather than by drugs, inhibiting the release of enzymes and so on. Expect your doctor to know something about some of these advances, or to be willing to find out on your behalf.
- Drugs deal with the results of disease, rarely the causes.
- Treat the patient, not the disease.
- To try to cure the body without involving the total person is like trying to start a car with a flat battery: no amount of polish on the chromium will work — you must have that essential spark of power.
- You must not only find the right therapy for your own needs, but also the right therapist: listen for the singer as well as to the song.
- Whatever and whoever you choose will cost money. How much depends on the therapist. One I know merely asks you to pay what you think the treatment is worth, or what you can afford, and she even accepts barter: I have helped to pay her

with new-laid free-range eggs and home-grown tomatoes. But how can you pay for anything so priceless as good health?

- Welcome, rather than reject.
- Be open to new ideas.
- Flexibility in your relationships may lead to flexibility in your hip.
- Don't be resigned: 'Do not go gentle into that good night'.
- Pain can be corrective to teach us lessons about ourselves, which we have earlier failed to learn.
- Boredom is the friend of disease.
- The occasional icecream is a pleasure, but it isn't daily bread.
- Whatever you eat, enjoy it with a good appetite.
- *The most miraculous miracle is the human body.*
- There are few quick miracles in any of these alternative therapies . . . but plenty of slow ones.